Exploring Clinical Communication in Asia

Bloomsbury Studies in Language and Healthcare

Series editors: Jack Pun and Dennis Tay

Providing a broad, up-to-date, comprehensive, and systematic overview of the latest research into language and healthcare, the *Bloomsbury Studies in Language and Healthcare* series explores the importance of interdisciplinary research to the fields of language, linguistics, communication, healthcare, and medicine.

Written by international researchers from a wide range of disciplines, including healthcare professionals, medical educators, linguists, and clinicians, books within the series offer a variety of perspectives and approaches. Cutting across the boundaries between linguistics and medicine, they investigate how communication affects the quality of care patients receive from health providers in different clinical settings, and how effective communication enhances our understanding of the challenges and expectations in healthcare worldwide.

Other titles in the series

Multimodal Approaches to Healthcare Communication Research, edited by Keiko Tsuchiya, Frank Coffey and Kyota Nakamura

Exploring Clinical Communication in Asia

Culture, Discipline, Best Practice and Clinicians' Voices in the Chinese Context

Jack Pun and Audrey Chan

BLOOMSBURY ACADEMIC
LONDON • NEW YORK • OXFORD • NEW DELHI • SYDNEY

BLOOMSBURY ACADEMIC
Bloomsbury Publishing Plc, 50 Bedford Square, London, WC1B 3DP, UK
Bloomsbury Publishing Inc, 1359 Broadway, New York, NY 10018, USA
Bloomsbury Publishing Ireland, 29 Earlsfort Terrace, Dublin 2, D02 AY28, Ireland

BLOOMSBURY, BLOOMSBURY ACADEMIC and the Diana logo are trademarks of Bloomsbury Publishing Plc

First published in Great Britain 2026

Cover design: Jade Barnett
Cover image © Vince Cavataio/Getty Images

A catalogue record for this book is available from the British Library.

A catalog record for this book is available from the Library of Congress.

ISBN: HB: 978-1-3502-9811-8
ePDF: 978-1-3502-9812-5
eBook: 978-1-3502-9813-2

Series: Bloomsbury Studies in Language and Healthcare

Typeset by Deanta Global Publishing Services, Chennai, India

Contents

Figures

Tables

Foreword

Effective communication in healthcare is not merely a matter of exchanging information; it is a crucial determinant of patient outcomes, trust and the quality of care. In an era where medical advancements continue to push the boundaries of what is possible, the ability of healthcare professionals to engage in clear, culturally sensitive and patient-centred communication remains paramount. Nowhere is this more evident than in the East Asian context, where linguistic diversity, cultural traditions and evolving medical practices intersect in complex ways.

This book is a unique contribution to the field of health communication research, providing a comprehensive overview of health communication research and practice in the Chinese context and a detailed discussion of the cultural differences between the East and the West. It sheds light on the nuanced ways in which clinicians, patients and caregivers navigate medical interactions in a multilingual and multicultural society, offering critical insights into the challenges and opportunities inherent in this dynamic field.

The authors have brought together a wealth of research and expertise to offer a detailed examination of clinical communication in Hong Kong and beyond. The book highlights the complexities of translanguaging in medical interactions, the adaptation of Western patient-centred communication models to East Asian healthcare settings and the impact of cultural philosophies on doctor-patient relationships. By drawing on cutting-edge empirical research, this volume makes a significant contribution to both academic discourse and practical applications in medical education and training.

This is a must-read for students, researchers and practitioners interested in healthcare communication, particularly those working in or studying the evolving landscapes of Asian healthcare systems. The insights provided in this book have the potential to shape clinical training, inform healthcare policy and ultimately enhance patient care across diverse settings.

I commend this book unreservedly.

Diana Slade
Professor and Director, Institute for Communication in Health Care
Australian National University

1

Introduction

What is effective clinical research in East Asian contexts?

In the past decade, the body of literature on healthcare communication in East Asian contexts has been growing. Pun et al. (2018) conducted a large-scale review of health professional-patient communication practices in Hong Kong, South Korea, Japan, Taiwan and Mainland China to analyse thirty-eight studies, which facilitated the understanding of how Asian-based researchers interpret medical encounters in their cultural contexts. As the need to improve healthcare services arises in East Asia, governments have been implementing healthcare reforms. Thus, the research on clinical communication in East Asia has been growing over the years. Many doctors, nurses, caretakers, researchers, as well as policymakers face the challenge of figuring out to what extent they can and should adopt Western patient-centred clinical philosophies (such as those embedded in Canadian, American, British and Australian healthcare systems) to East Asian reforms on a daily basis. Acknowledging such a barrier, researchers have been dedicated to training clinicians to communicate effectively and achieve the full implementation of patient-centred care effectively in real-life practices.

The growing concern about effective communication in real-life clinical contexts reflects East Asian governments' aim of meeting the increasing demand for quality healthcare services by introducing healthcare reforms. As stated, it is crucial to learn how clinicians can appropriate Western patient-centred healthcare philosophies and apply them to non-English speaking contexts. For instance, during the standardised training of pre- and post-qualification clinicians in English-dominant settings, medical educators tend to use established models and texts like the Calgary-Cambridge Guides to teach healthcare communication skills (Kurtz & Silverman, 1996). On the other hand, there are no existing equivalent models for non-English-dominant settings. Very limited work has also been attempted to translate Western models of communication for clinicians working in East Asian contexts. Moreover, a limited amount of research has studied the differences in clinical communication between English and non-English settings (Claramita et al., 2013; Slade et al., 2015a; 2015b; Pun et al., 2016a; 2016b), making it inappropriate for medical educators to directly adopt the desired Western model in non-English speaking contexts.

While clinicians in East Asian contexts and their counterparts in English-speaking settings both encounter mutual barriers such as time pressures, high patient loads, high patient expectations and pressure from management, increasingly improved patient health literacy, pressure to build trusting physician/nurse-patient relationships and different socio-cultural elements result in various cultural-specific barriers. To help the reader understand the variations of clinical communication barriers between different cultures, this book focuses on the case of Hong Kong. It offers the reader an insight into multilingual issues as medical professionals are trained in English while they verbally talk to their patients in the patient's native language, Cantonese (Seijo et al., 1991; Erzinger, 1991; Slade et al., 2015a; 2015b). It is crucial to emphasise that the clinical settings of Hong Kong are very different from that of mainland China as the city has two official languages, namely Chinese (including the two spoken varieties of Cantonese and Mandarin, and standard written Chinese) and English (Evans, 2010). More than seven million of the inhabitants are native speakers of Cantonese (Pun, 2021a; 2021b). Thus, Cantonese has remained the dominant vernacular cum lingua franca in the city. English is usually perceived as a prestige language in many local contexts, particularly in educational settings, and is the most widely used medium for tertiary teaching (Pun, 2021). Therefore, people living in Hong Kong often code-switch between Cantonese and English. Simultaneously, the use of Mandarin is rocketing as there is an increasing number of non-Cantonese Chinese visitors and residents immigrating to Hong Kong. People who do not have adequate communication skills in the local languages often require help from interpreters during crucial occasions such as hospital appointments. Their lack of knowledge of the local languages leads to their incapability to express themselves accurately and efficiently (Pun, 2021). In local healthcare contexts, although the majority of clinicians are bilingual and native speakers of Cantonese, they are taught in English in medical schools (Pun, 2021). This implies that they are usually unfamiliar with Chinese medical terminology. When performing their daily tasks, they read and record nearly the entirety of their patients' medical records in the form of written English but orally speak with their patients in Cantonese. They also often code-switch or practise translanguaging with their colleagues in spoken Cantonese mixed with medical

English. More and more research projects in the recent decade have strived to develop frameworks to achieve effective clinical handover using standardised communication protocols, including the Identify, Situation, Background, Assessment and Recommendation (ISBAR) protocol (Finnigan et al., 2010; Femming & Hübner, 2013; Kitney et al., 2016; Robertson et al., 2014), where the stated protocol has been proven to be useful in organising handover steps and thus minimising the chances of miscommunication and misunderstanding between healthcare providers. However, not enough attention has been paid to the use of translanguaging in clinical communication. Clearly, publications on the influences of translanguaging on medical handovers are lacking, with just Pun et al. (2019a; 2019b) examining the use of Connect, Ask, Respond and Empathise (CARE) protocol in a local bilingual hospital.

With that in mind, by studying the clinical contexts in Hong Kong, especially in terms of the use of translanguaging, this book gains insights from the area of interactional sociolinguistics, which helps the researchers understand the micro details of multilingual interactions and contextual contexts in which the medical encounters are carried out to learn how social goals are achieved (Demjén, 2016) in East Asian societies and multicultural settings. Drawing on socially oriented functional linguistics, this study offers a detailed and systematic overview of the role that language plays in clinician-patient communication in East Asian contexts. Audio/video recordings of clinician-patient communication, semi-structured interviews and ethnographic observations comprise data for the research. Using a cross-disciplinary approach combining the expertise of linguists, clinicians and health communication researchers, the contributing authors identify communication features of effective and ineffective interactions, focusing on the communication breakdowns and vulnerable points which jeopardise the quality and safety of the patient experience. This book aims to develop a specific culturally appropriate communication model and to provide detailed and research-driven recommendations for healthcare professionals, which may ultimately improve therapeutic relationships and ensure patient safety. While the model in this book is developed within a particular socio-cultural and medical context, it is our hope that it will be modified and adapted further afield and contribute to a deeper understanding of actual communicative practices where clinicians engage in different clinical encounters. Building on cutting-edge empirical research on the health communication landscape in Asia, this book addresses topics of interest to researchers in health communication and applied linguistics in general. It also provides healthcare professionals with the resources necessary for a critical reflection of their professional practice. Insights can inform communication training programmes for practising healthcare professionals and medical students.

Researching East Asian health communication: A translational approach

As stated, current Western models are not entirely suitable for the delivery of clinical services in East Asia. Recognising this research gap, my colleagues and I adopt a unique methodological approach – translational communication research – which directly addresses real-world healthcare communication challenges. This approach integrates investigative concepts, expertise, tools and methodologies from various disciplines to produce practical, evidence-based outcomes that benefit both healthcare users and providers (Eggins & Slade, 2015). Our study employs an ethnographic discourse approach, analysing clinician-patient interactions to assess communication quality and identify discourse strategies used by doctors or nurses to engage with their patients. Specifically, we analyse interview transcripts and clinical encounters with healthcare professionals from a diverse range of specialties, including intensive care, oncology, neurology, surgery, geriatrics, nursing, palliative care, obstetrics and gynaecology, and traditional Chinese medicine. These professionals bring a range of medical experience from early-career physicians to senior practitioners with over fifteen years of clinical experience.

The data collection process included semi-structured interviews and direct field observations. The interviews, conducted over a period of six months, ranged from 60 to 120 minutes per session, approximately 30 hours of recorded dialogue. These conversations provided insights into clinicians' perspectives on patient communication, challenges they face and the strategies they employ. Additionally, we conducted on-site ethnographic fieldwork in hospital wards and outpatient clinics, where we observed real-time clincian-patient interactions to contextualise our findings. This multi-method approach enhances the validity of our study by capturing both self-reported experiences and naturally occurring discourse in clinical settings. By analysing these rich data sources, each chapter in this volume unpacks the complexities of clinical communication in different clinical settings. The findings contribute to evidence-based recommendations for an effective communication model that enhances patient engagement, minimises misunderstandings and ultimately improves the quality and safety of healthcare services, mitigating the risks of undesirable clinical outcomes.

To ensure a clear and logical presentation of our findings, the book is structured into two main sections. *Part I: Insights from Interviews with Doctors* (Chapters 2 to 9) presents original research drawn from interviews and clinical observations, offering first-hand perspectives on communication strategies employed across various medical specialties. *Part II: Skills for Effective Clinical Communication* (Chapters 10 to 12) consists of review papers and original research, synthesising key findings and best practices to enhance clinician-patient interactions. This structured approach allows for a comprehensive exploration of healthcare communication, integrating both empirical research and practical insights to inform future clinical practice.

The studies included in this book were conducted by a cross-disciplinary research team from the fields of Nursing, Linguistics, Medicine and Communication. Building on existing collaborations in Hong Kong and in Australia, our team has been conducting research and training for nurses and doctors about effective clinical communication. We had been working in collaboration with both public hospitals (Hospital Authority in Hong Kong) and private hospitals in developing professional training for effective clinical communication since 2010. The team focused on the unique Asian aspects of health communication in Hong Kong as the system traverses a unique mix of Western and Chinese values, serving as a comparative basis for evaluating cross-cultural expectations, practices and experiences between East and West. The complex sociolinguistic reality riddled with multilingualism poses considerable challenges to clinical communication. Our researchers move from collecting qualitative discourse data to delivering training and reflection sessions with clinicians in Chinese settings.

This book explores the development of effective clinical communication by bridging research insights from both Eastern and Western contexts. It consists of thirteen chapters on reporting the latest research in various settings of health communication such as doctor-patient interactions, nurse handovers and cross-disciplinary communication to provide a broad, comprehensive overview of the complexity and heterogeneity of health communication in the Chinese context, which is gradually moving beyond a preference for Western-based models to one that considers the local culture in understanding and interpreting medical encounters.

The introductory chapter establishes the book's central theme and underscores the significance of effective clinical communication within Chinese healthcare contexts. It outlines the historical development and evolution of clinical communication research, drawing comparisons between Western and Eastern models of healthcare interaction. In doing so, it critically examines key studies and findings from both global and regional perspectives, positioning Hong Kong's multilingual healthcare setting as a case study to illustrate the complex interplay of cultural and linguistic diversity in medical encounters. This chapter also introduces the book's structure and research objectives, providing an overview of the chapters that follow while emphasising the practical and theoretical contributions of the research.

Part I: Insights from interviews with doctors

The first section presents empirical research based on interviews with doctors across a range of medical specialties. Chapter 2 offers a review of healthcare communication research in East Asia, with a particular focus on the cultural and linguistic influences that shape clinician-patient interactions. It examines key themes, including family-centred decision-making, traditional Chinese philosophical perspectives on health and mortality, and patient expectations regarding clinical engagement. This chapter critically evaluates existing literature, identifies gaps in the field and contextualises the research questions that guide the subsequent chapters.

The chapters (Chapters 3 to 9) that follow present findings from the interviews with practitioners in clinical fields such as oncology,palliative care, neurology, surgery, nursing, geriatric care and veterinary medicine. Drawing on semi-structured interviews, these chapters analyse how healthcare professionals navigate the challenges of clinical communication in both primary care and hospital settings. They examine how power relations, cultural values and language proficiency affect communication strategies, particularly in high-stakes interactions such as breaking bad news, discussing end-of-life care, obtaining informed consent and negotiating treatment plans. The book also explores the intersection of Western and Traditional Chinese Medicine, with Chapter 11, which focuses on communication in Traditional Chinese Medicine consultations, now repositioned earlier in the section to align with discussions on culturally specific models of patient-centred care.

Each chapter functions as a case study, presenting real-life examples of clinical communication through detailed transcripts and narratives from practising doctors. These accounts illustrate how clinicians manage different stages of patient interaction, including history-taking, diagnosis, treatment discussions and end-of-life decision-making. The analysis extends to the interpersonal and ethical dimensions of clinical communication, addressing how clinicians engage with patients and their families while navigating institutional constraints and cultural expectations. Through such discussion, the book highlights recurring themes in medical discourse, such as the role of metaphors in patient counselling, the negotiation of medical authority in cross-cultural consultations and the emotional labour involved in delivering sensitive information. The inclusion of authentic clinical anecdotes and interview excerpts provides researchers with a comprehensive understanding of the communication practices that define contemporary medical encounters in East Asia.

Part II: Skills for effective clinical communication

The second section shifts from empirical research to the practical application of communication strategies in clinical settings. This part of the book builds on the findings presented in Part I and explores ways for improving communication in specialised areas such as critical care medicine (i.e. EDs and ICUs), primary care and clinical handovers. The discussion examines the communicative challenges inherent in high-risk environments, focusing on how clinicians manage time constraints, patient anxiety and institutional hierarchies in fast-paced medical settings. The book also considers the implications of advocating for a 'speak-up' culture in Chinese medical institutions, where traditional power structures often discourage open dialogue between junior and senior staff.

The chapters in this section further analyse the role of communication in primary care, addressing the difficulties clinicians face in building rapport and fostering patient trust in culturally diverse settings. This discussion extends to the specific case of nursing handovers, where effective communication is essential for ensuring patient safety. The analysis considers the impact of structured handover protocols, technological advancements, and language proficiency on the efficiency and accuracy of information transfer. The book also explores the role of patient involvement in the handover process, assessing how communication strategies can be adapted to facilitate more inclusive and transparent medical discussions.

The concluding chapter synthesises the key themes presented throughout the book, emphasising the unique characteristics of medical communication in East Asian contexts. It revisits the role of power dynamics in clinician-patient relationships and highlights the ways in which cultural and linguistic factors influence medical discourse. The discussion extends to interdisciplinary communication challenges, particularly in multilingual clinical environments such as Hong Kong, where medical professionals must navigate both professional hierarchies and language barriers. The final section also considers the broader implications of these findings for clinical practice, medical education and healthcare policy. It proposes strategies for implementing culturally appropriate patient-centred care in East Asia, advocating for institutional changes that support more effective communication training for clinicians. The book concludes with recommendations for future research, suggesting areas for further exploration in the study of clinical communication in multilingual and multicultural medical settings.

To conclude, the research presented in this book highlights the complexities of clinical communication in East Asian contexts, where cultural, linguistic and institutional factors shape healthcare interactions in ways distinct from Western models. The multilingual and multicultural environment of Hong Kong, as one of the foci of study, underscores the challenges and opportunities in adapting patient-centred communication frameworks to settings where medical education, documentation and interaction occur across multiple languages. Understanding these contextual nuances is crucial for refining communication strategies that enhance patient trust, improve health outcomes and align with culturally specific expectations of care. Building on this foundation, the next chapter critically examines existing research on healthcare communication in Asia. It explores how cultural values – such as family-oriented decision-making, Confucian philosophies of care and perceptions of a 'good death' – shape medical encounters. By identifying knowledge gaps and recurrent challenges in clinical communication, the next chapter lays the groundwork for developing a model of patient-centred care that integrates both Western and Eastern communication styles.

Part I

Insights from interviews with clinicians

2

Healthcare communication research from the East

This chapter reviews former relevant studies of healthcare communication in Asia, with a focus on the cultural factors in understanding and interpreting medical encounters against this contextual background, including family-oriented, Chinese philosophies that define effective communication and the concept of good death. It critically evaluates these previous studies, identifies existing knowledge gaps, presents the research questions and argues for the need to conduct the current research. It critically reviews and discusses a number of re-occurring health communication issues in Asia context research that constitute the broad field of clinical communication such as power and relationship among healthcare providers, patients and their families as well as cultural attitudes, communication preferences that influence decision-making and patient satisfaction. It then investigates how a Chinese model of patient-centred care should be built by merging the communication styles of Traditional Chinese Medicine (TCM) practitioners. It further discusses the rise of health literacy of patients in the Chinese context that has led to an explosion of online health resources and pharmaceutical company products, which have profoundly affected the way in which healthcare is delivered. This has brought about changes in the dynamics and power between healthcare providers and their patients.

Cultural influences: How to interpret Eastern medical communication?

Eastern expectations and issues in doctor- and nurse-patient interactions: Emotional support, authorial communicative patterns and sexism

As per cross-disciplinary studies, Asian patients tend to focus more on physical comfort rather than the emotional support offered by medical service providers, nurses in particular (Jiang et al., 2015). Based on a caring nurse-patient communication scale, Jiang et al.'s study showed that nurses were better at offering operative care, including utilising specialised equipment and implementing medical treatments. Contrarily, Chinese nurses had difficulties demonstrating care to their patients, meaning that they lacked the skills of showing empathetic attitudes and building rapport as well as trust. Pun et al. (2018) later compared Jiang et al.'s study (2015) to Dong et al.'s research on Chinese terminal cancer patients, which proved that nurses took up the responsibility of offering their patients physical comfort while doctors treated patients' symptoms and managed their rights (Dong et al., 2016). As per Liu et al. (2005), Chinese healthcare contexts are unlike Western ones because healthcare providers have particular cultural approaches to dealing with illness and misfortune. As a result, bad news delivery is considered a private and familial matter, thus excluding nurses in the process of carrying out challenging conversations (Liu et al., 2005). In addition to that, since Chinese people consider death as a subject of taboo, there is a need for nurses to develop culturally appropriate communication strategies to interact with cancer patients in Chinese settings (Pun et al., 2018).

Doctor-patient power dynamics are also essentially different in the East as the relationships between the two parties are asymmetrical (Ishikawa & Yamazaki, 2005). According to Wang (2010), Chinese patients have a preference for their doctors to play the dominant role when compared to American patients. This thus results in doctor-centred interactions, leading to patients' dissatisfaction as there is often a long waiting time for very short medical consultations (Yin et al., 2012). This cultural influence has led to other negative patient experiences as well. For example, when seeing their male urologists for their overactive bladders, Hong Kong female patients feel embarrassed to explain their symptoms and often have no choice when planning their treatments (Siu, 2015). Just as Hsiao et al. (2006) explained, the conventional role of men in Chinese societies had made male practitioners show less empathy (Hsiao et al., 2006) because patriarchal ideologies discouraged men to express themselves, thus resulting in poor communication (Attree, 2001). Kim et al. (2008) also pointed out the problems that arise during the communication of sexual history in the East: 25 per cent of the interviewed patients in their study experienced negative emotions when telling their male doctors about their sexual concerns. These studies have demonstrated and problematised the role of patriarchy in forming hierarchical Eastern doctor-patient relationships, demonstrating the need for male doctors and female patients in particular to foster better communication.

A family-based communication model and its collectivist power dynamics

In the area of clinical interactions in the East, the model of family-based communication is a recurring and crucial theme. In traditional Chinese societies, patients' families are often considered the key decision-makers regarding patients' treatments. Lin et al. (2016) observed that patients were often unwilling or unable to express their discomfort directly with practitioners. Instead, their families gave informed consent on their behalf, deciding what would be the most suitable options in terms of treatments, reflecting a less affiliated, controlled, doctor-domination communication tendency in Chinese societies, paralleling Confucian values (Cong, 2004).

That being said, not all Chinese medical settings are alike. For example, Hong Kong is a culturally diverse city, implicating the opportunity of integrating elements from Western patient-centred models (Pun et al., 2018). Unlike mainland Chinese patients, Wong et al. stressed the feasibility of planning an advanced directive with advanced malignancy with Hong Kong patients (Wong et al., 2012). To do so, doctors should engage pro-actively with their patients on their end-of-life (EOL) arrangements (Wong et al., 2012). They are encouraged to form mutual goals with their patients and family members; therefore, the patients can be involved in the decision-making stage (Wong et al., 2012). Recent research results in Japan have also demonstrated an increasing trend for medical providers to involve their patients in decision-making processes. Scholars based in Japan noted that nurses were requested to look for medical/care solutions based on the Japanese values of respect and harmony (Konishi et al., 2009; Konishi & Davis, 1999), thus intervening and reconciling the relationship between patients and their family members (Toda et al., 2015). Therefore, the clinical research in Hong Kong and Japan has suggested the value of integrating Western patient-centred models with Eastern cultural values and thus stressed the need for more cross-cultural studies on the points of convergence between Eastern and Western clinical communication models.

Aiding patients to have a 'good death'

Many research projects conducted in the English-speaking world have extensively studied EOL communication. However, studies of similar nature that investigate Asian EOL conversations are lacking. The clinical contexts in the East embody very different beliefs and practices, especially when considering

EOL care, compared to those in English-speaking countries. Most significantly, Chinese people believe in the idea of having a 'good death'. They think that the act of talking about death brings bad luck. This makes Chinese families unwilling to talk about EOL matters and medical service providers hesitant about informing their dying patients of relevant prognoses (Pun et al., 2021a). However, it brings more benefits to patients and their families if doctors feel comfortable and safe to carry out honest conversations with them to discuss treatment expectations, dying wishes and barriers they may encounter (Wright et al., 2008), which in turn allows the happenings of 'good deaths' (Pun et al., 2021). Otherwise, ineffective EOL communication may lead to negative results including aggressive life-sustaining care, insufficient focus on patients' well-being and sabotaging the quality of patients' care (Pun et al., 2021).

Cultural attitudes that build and shape trust, decision-making and patient satisfaction

As per Pun et al. (2015a), patients' level of trust in their doctors varies according to their level of satisfaction with medical services and conversations (Pun et al., 2015), particularly in Hong Kong. Lee et al. (2013) also found that more satisfying primary outcomes would be generated if South Korean patients had known primary care doctors for a relatively longer period (Lee et al., 2013). In Taiwan, hospital complaints also often plummet when healthcare providers and their patients are both more active in conversations (Zhang et al., 2011). Patients and their families' attitudes towards practitioners and associated hospitals usually determine the decisions of filing malpractice lawsuits (Zhang et al., 2011).

Pun et al. (2018) further explored varying degrees of patients' expectations in terms of the levels of involvement during decision-making processes across Asian regions. For example, as stated, Mainland Chinese patients often opt for a more doctor-dominant mode of communication, while Hong Kong patients like to be more active in medical encounters (Pun et al., 2018). Zhang et al. (2011) similarly observed that most Mainland Chinese patients normally played a passive role during decision-making processes (Zhang et al., 2011). On the other hand, Hong Kong patients would actively prioritise and stress their needs while acknowledging their practitioners' expertise simultaneously (Henderson & Chien, 2007), possibly because of Hong Kong people's emphasis on reassurance, patient confidentiality and individualist values (Arthur et al., 2004). Contrarily, while South Korea is also in East Asia, its core Confucian societal values make doctor-patient relationships in the country similar to those in China. South

Korean practitioners tend to demonstrate less empathy when talking to their patients (Kim et al., 2008). Noh et al. (2009) study also found that less than half of the Korean women suffering from cervical cancer would actively seek information on their illness as they had the need to learn more.

These research studies together have outlined the influences of traditional cultural traditions on patient participation and how these traditions could lead to patients' unwillingness to share their medical history or ask their doctors for more information regarding their conditions (Cong, 2004). Therefore, the level of patient involvement during decision-making processes remains the most significant determinant of patient satisfaction, like how often they would feel welcomed to discuss medical issues with their doctors and how accessible the practitioners could be when having to disclose danger symptoms regarding their illnesses and treatments when getting discharged from the hospitals (Pun et al., 2018).

In practice: Building the Chinese model of patient-centred care in Hong Kong

In Hong Kong, the Hospital Authority, the governing body that is in charge of the management of local public hospitals, has established the model of patient-centred care as the key value for the delivery of medical with the implementation of a communicative direction of effective 'two-way communication' as 'indispensable for understanding and meeting a patient's needs' (Hong Kong Hospital Authority, 2013). However, the model is not deemed fully suitable for local medical settings as critical incidents occur quite frequently and patients feel dissatisfied (Griffiths & Yeoh, 2011) because of inefficient clinician-patient, clinician-clinician communication (Hong Kong Hospital Authority, 2014). Practitioners in Hong Kong tend to pay more attention to their patients' physical needs than their social and emotional needs, making the patients feel that the doctors are deprioritising their care in hospital wards (Pun et al., 2018). Pun et al. (2016a) found a similar pattern among local nurses since they were more attentive to their actions than the interpersonal dimension of care delivery.

Aiming to tackle such issues and improve local patients' impressions of medical care, Pun et al. (2018) suggested some useful practices for medical service providers to implement effective patient-centred communication.

To explore Hong Kong patients' perception of good medical practice in terms ofhealth communication, the research team conducted interdisciplinary research on the field of communication along with observations of medical scenes. For example, small gestures such as smiling, laughter, affective body language, aiding patients to fulfil simple wishes and demonstrating sincere attitudes can show the patients that the healthcare workers are sensitive to their needs and thus care about them (Yam & Rossiter, 2000). Zayts and Kang (2010) also emphasised that information delivery must be interactive when healthcare workers face patients' initial inquiries. They also found it important for doctors to attend to both their patients' treatment plans and psycho-social needs, which allows them to offer holistic and integral medical care. Moreover, clinicians are encouraged to be empathetic and caring in the stages of diagnoses and treatments (Zayts & Kang, 2010).

These insights from Hong Kong-based research have also shed light on the rising trend of patient-centred care in East Asia in general. In Japan, for instance, medical consultations are usually rather short while physical examinations as well as diagnostic explanations are longer when compared to those in the United States, which leads to patient dissatisfaction (Ohtaki et al., 2003). Goto et al. (2015) also found that Japanese patients are generally more satisfied with their doctors when they feel that the doctors are willing to listen to their stories. These doctors tend to engage with their patients more actively when noting their medical history and diagnosing (Goto et al., 2015). Takayama et al. (2001) also observed that patients would be less likely to experience anxiety even when they are informed of negative examination results if they are happy with their doctors' communicative styles. Therefore, there is an increasing need for East Asian healthcare workers to be trained to employ effective communication skills when interacting with patients.

Learning from TCM communication styles

It is also useful to learn from TCM practitioners' communication styles as TCM tends to offer patients more interpersonal support when compared to the context of Western medicine (WM) because the practitioners demonstrate better communication skills (Zhang & Sleeboom-Faulkner, 2011). Compared to patients receiving treatments in WM contexts, those in TCM settings show higher patient satisfaction in general because they perceive their TCM practitioners as better listeners (Chung et al., 2009). Chan (1995) and Zhou and Nunes (2012) also observed that TCM practitioners seem to be more attentive to their patients' personal experiences and have a more comprehensive overview of how a patient's physical body relates to the whole system (Chan, 1995; Chung et al., 2009).

For WM doctors to learn from TCM doctors, they must first understand the differences and similarities between the philosophies that define the consultations in the two contexts (Gu, 1999; Jin, 2018). TCM patients believe that TCM is based on Confucius values (Zhou & Nunes, 2012). TCM practitioners also express a variety of ways to treat their patients, unlike the narrow range observed among WM doctors (Zhou & Nunes, 2012). TCM practitioners often prioritise listening to their patients' personal experiences as it allows them to achieve a more holistic overview of the interactions between the physical body and the surroundings instead of merely the illnesses or physical symptoms (Chan, 1995; Zhou & Nunes, 2012). TCM practitioners use the five examination skills of *wang4* (i.e. looking at visible symptoms), *wen2* (examining the patient's voice, heartbeat and odour in the oral cavity), *wen2* (asking the patient about their symptoms and medical history), *qie4* (examining pulse) and *zhen4* (making diagnoses) (Gu, 1999). These steps allow the practitioners to attend to their patients' interpersonal and emotional needs more closely (Zhang & Sleeboom-Faulkner, 2011).

By being good listeners to their patients, TCM practitioners prioritise interpersonal matters over physical discomfort, thus enhancing their patients' compliance with their planned treatments and knowledge of their body conditions. Therefore, TCM patients mostly cooperate better in terms of the modification of their biomedical behaviours, leading to more positive clinical outcomes. On the other hand, WM patients are more likely to be not happy with the quality of medical interactions with their practitioners (Chung et al., 2009). These studies have demonstrated that it is essential for doctors to acquire excellent listening skills in order to establish trusting doctor-patient relationships and thus speed up patients' recovery process as they cooperate with their doctors to identify the causes of their illnesses and plan appropriate treatments accordingly. The role of doctor-patient communication has been proven to be extremely crucial in cross-cultural medical encounters. It can affect medical outcomes including patient satisfaction and compliance, complaints, medical litigation, symptom resolution as well as pain control (Taylor et al., 2002; Dowsett et al., 2000; Vincent et al., 1995).

WM doctors are encouraged to learn from TCM practitioners in terms of understanding their patients' needs holistically in order to better the rate of patient compliance. It is useful to consider patients' interpersonal needs alongside their physical concerns (Vincent et al., 1995). The unique way of building interpersonal rapport in TCM settings (Lu et al., 2004; Chung et al., 2009; Wang, 2010) allows practitioners to have a better understanding of their patients' interpersonal problems and physical discomfort, and help the patients learn about their medical conditions as well as modify their daily habits, leading to subsequently more desirable long-term medical outcomes (Pun, 2020). When considering an intercultural medical context like Hong Kong, it is thus important for researchers and healthcare providers to understand how cross-cultural elements may be utilised to facilitate medical communication (Slade et al., 2015b; Ribeiro & Hoyle, 2009; Gu, 1999).

Improving health literacy in the East

While a lot of studies have demonstrated that patients' knowledge of hospice and palliative care is one of the key elements relevant to the completion of advanced directives (AD), a limited amount of research has investigated the role of health literacy in East Asian patients' willingness to be part of the planning stage of advance care (Bazargan et al., 2021; Bazargan & Bazargan-Hejazi, 2021; Nouri et al., 2019; Stuart, 2017).

By improving health literacy in the population, patients have more knowledge of illnesses and the concept of Ads, which in turn motivates them to plan their own care (Chen & Weng, 2023) as they become more competent in accessing, learning, appraising and applying acquired health information to make better judgements and decisions on their treatments (Sørensen et al., 2013).

Berkman et al.'s (2011) systematic review indicated that poor health literacy leads to a lot of undesirable medical outcomes, including diabetes, sexually transmitted illnesses, dental problems as well as cardiovascular diseases. People with low health literacy also tend to be quite passive when looking for health information (Berkman et al., 2011) and less willing to communicate with healthcare providers (Katz et al., 2007). They rarely actively discuss their ideas when making shared decisions (Smith et al., 2013). They would rather let their doctors make decisions on their behalf (Smithers et al., 2018), aligning with the general trend in East Asian medical settings. Therefore, it is significant to promote health literacy in order to help patients understand, complete and use advance directives timely (Chen et al., 2022). Considering how much cultural, religious as well as personal values impact patients' EOL decisions in Asia (Chen & Weng, 2023), it is essential to increase health literacy. Patients will be able to make informed EOL decisions as they can understand medical terms, what life-sustaining treatments may lead to, and express their communicating preferences to their doctors and nurses (Nutbeam, 2000). It also facilitates the collaboration between family members and healthcare workers when making future healthcare decisions in collectivist settings (Chen & Weng, 2023).

*

This chapter has reviewed a wide range of studies on healthcare communication in Asia, highlighting the impact of cultural values, communication preferences and patient expectations in shaping medical interactions. By identifying key features of cross-cultural communication and the unique needs of patients in various regions – especially Hong Kong – this chapter has provided insights into how Western medicine (WM) healthcare professionals can adapt their practices to align with local expectations. In particular, it is crucial for doctors and nurses to recognise the collectivist, family-centred nature of healthcare decision-making and patients' often passive roles in medical consultations. As a result, healthcare professionals must enhance their attentiveness to patients' emotional and interpersonal needs, mirroring the communication approaches of Traditional Chinese Medicine (TCM) practitioners. This understanding can also contribute to the promotion of better health literacy and improved patient-provider relationships.

Building on these themes, the next chapter explores communication practices within TCM, offering a deeper examination of how its holistic, patient-centred approach fosters trust and long-term therapeutic relationships. By analysing discourse patterns and practitioner-patient interactions, Chapter 3 will provide insights into how communication strategies in TCM can inform and enhance patient care across different medical settings.

3

Traditional Chinese medicine

TCM Practitioners' insights into the holistic approach to communication

Building trusting relationships between Traditional Chinese Medicine (TCM) practitioners and patients

In recent decades, TCM has gained increasing popularity and attention within global medical settings. TCM practitioners are trained to address their patients' health issues based on a holistic approach, placing an emphasis on the integrity of the human body and its close relationship with both its social and natural environments. Physiologically, TCM theories view the body through systematic analysis and cybernetic methods (Lu et al., 2004). Applying the natural diagnostic approach of 'Zheng', TCM practitioners strive to understand their patients' conditions. Building on such understanding, the practitioners perform an in-depth examination of the concerned conditions and signs, including imbalances in pulse, energy or life force, and organ function (Chan, 1995).

In contrast to Western medicine (WM), TCM emphasises a comprehensive assessment of several bodily systems as well as organs and places greater value on the patient's personal experiences. TCM pracititioners aim to gain a complete picture of the patient's physical and environmental factors. However, WM focuses on identifying the underlying causes of illness through scientific analysis (Zhou & Nunes, 2012). WM doctors use advanced medical equipment to perform examinations and rely on data-driven diagnoses (Chung et al., 2009). Consultations in WM tend to focus on explaining diagnostic results, whereas TCM employs four key diagnostic methods: inspection, auscultation and olfaction (listening and smelling), inquiry, and palpation, known collectively as si-zhen, to identify and diagnose illnesses (Chan, 1995).

Like WM doctors, TCM doctors prescribe treatments after a thorough analysis based on their reflections after going through these four diagnostic methods.

That being said, TCM patients typically continue seeing the same practitioner over multiple visits, fostering long-term care and strong practitioner-patient relationships. This contrasts with the less consistent care in Hong Kong's WM system, where patients often seek different doctors. Continuous relationships in TCM are believed to be helpful to the enhancement of clinical outcomes, the process of shared decision-making and the improvement of patient satisfaction (Wang, 2010). Over the last few years, TCM has become more integrated into Hong Kong's healthcare system, leading to an increase in patients combining TCM with WM treatments (Chung et al., 2009). Nonetheless, research on the impact of TCM practices on WM treatments remains limited (Lu et al., 2004).

In response to this research gap, this chapter presents a study examining practitioner-patient interactions within Hong Kong's TCM primary care context. The study was the first to explore TCM communication in a local Cantonese environment, analysing ten authentic consultations between TCM practitioners and their patients. Through these interviews, the study explored the nature and communication style of TCM consultations and identified typical stages of discourse in such encounters.

To gain a comprehensive understanding of how TCM practitioners and patients collaboratively construct biomedical knowledge and achieve a shared interpretation of the patient's condition, this study employs discourse analysis approach. The transcripts included in this chapter were drawn from a previous study (Pun et al., 2017); however, the analysis and interpretations have been further developed to align with the focus of this chapter. The findings highlighted the role of 'touch' – a term describing the holistic nature of TCM consultations – as a key aspect of developing therapeutic relationships based on Chinese cultural practices. The research identified numerous linguistic strategies TCM practitioners use to provide patient-centred care and support shared decision-making. These approaches were found to be effective in improving patient comprehension and adherence to treatment (Pun, 2020). The study also suggested ways to improve the quality of patient experiences during TCM consultations.

Interpersonal support

Recent research suggests that TCM provides patients with stronger interpersonal support compared to WM, as TCM practitioners tend to be more skilled in communication (Zhang & Sleeboom-Faulkner, 2011). Chung et al. (2009) also examined medical communication and patient perceptions in both TCM and WM settings, finding that patient satisfaction is often higher in TCM. This was largely due to patients perceiving TCM practitioners as better listeners. Chan (1995) and Zhou and Nunes (2012) noted that TCM doctors focus more on the patient's personal experiences and take a more comprehensive view when considering how the patient's body relates to the broader system (Chan, 1995; Chung et al., 2009).

Past comparative studies of TCM and WM interactions highlighted numerous differences and some similarities in the philosophies that form the basis of the consultations (Gu, 1999; Jin, 2018; Xu & Yang, 2009). Some evidence indicated that patients might prefer a passive communication style and even associate TCM with Confucian values. Other studies found that various TCM practitioners approach patient care very differently, while WM doctors show a more uniform approach (Zhou & Nunes, 2012). In TCM, doctors often focus on personal experiences, aiming for a holistic understanding of the connection between the body and the environment rather than focusing solely on symptoms or illnesses (Chan, 1995; Zhou & Nunes, 2012). TCM doctors assess their patients using five diagnostic methods: observing visible signs ('wang4'); examining the voice, heartbeat and oral cavity odour ('wen2'); asking about symptoms and medical history ('wen2'); checking the pulse ('qie4'); and finally diagnosing ('zhen4') (Gu, 1999). Studies in countries where TCM supports primary care services suggested that TCM practitioners provide greater emotional and interpersonal support compared to their WM counterparts (Zhang & Sleeboom-Faulkner, 2011). In a large-scale study conducted in the United States, participating patients noted that TCM practitioners' communication skills were more appreciated than those of their general practitioners (Jin & Tay, 2017).

By focusing on their patients' interpersonal issues in addition to physical symptoms, TCM doctors are more likely to persuade their patients to comply with the recommended treatments and help them understand their own health. This leads to better patient cooperation in making changes to their biomedical behaviours, resulting in improved clinical outcomes. Chung et al. (2009) found that WM patients were more frequently dissatisfied with their interactions with doctors. Jagosh et al. (2011) also highlighted the importance of strong listening skills in building positive doctor-patient relationships, which aid the recovery process by helping doctors identify illness causes and determine the best treatments.

Previous studies also emphasised the significance of exploring cross-cultural aspects of practitioner-patient communication. Effective interactions between doctors and patients can influence medical outcomes such as patient satisfaction and adherence, complaints, symptom relief, pain management and even medical litigation (Taylor et al., 2002; Dowsett et al., 2000; Ong et al., 2000; Vincent et al., 1995; Stewart, 1995).

Recent research suggested that understanding both the interpersonal and physical needs of patients is crucial to encouraging compliance with treatment decisions. This is due to the consideration of their broader interpersonal concerns alongside physical health issues (Vincent et al., 1995; Stewart, 1995). TCM settings are noted for their unique development of interpersonal rapport (Lu et al., 2004; Chung et al., 2009; Wang, 2010). By addressing both interpersonal and physical matters, TCM practitioners enhance patient compliance, promote greater self-awareness of health conditions and facilitate the adoption of healthier habits, contributing to better long-term outcomes compared to WM patients (Pun, 2020). Although clinical communication research in Hong Kong has become more and more common, the existing scholarship mainly focuses on WM contexts (Slade et al., 2015b; Ribeiro & Hoyle, 2009; Gu, 1999). Hence, this chapter aims to offer a starting point for researchers to further close the gap.

Si-zhen: Wàng, wén, wèn and *qiè* as patient-centred examination

In Western countries, especially in the United States, the idea of patient-centred care has gained widespread popularity. This approach has also become a key policy within Hong Kong's hospital system. Research has identified specific strategies for providing patient-centred care in primary healthcare settings. For effective implementation in Hong Kong, active doctor participation is considered crucial, because patients often prefer their physicians to take on an authoritative role (Ho & Koenig, 2014). While Western medicine tends to focus primarily on illnesses or symptoms, TCM takes a holistic view, considering the patient's overall life, body and environment (Chan, 1995; Zhou & Nunes, 2012). As a result, TCM and WM evaluate patients in fundamentally different ways. In TCM, practitioners use the four diagnostic methods: wàng 望 (observation through looking), wén 聞(listening and smelling), wèn 問(inquiry) and qiè 切 (pulse analysis), whereas Western doctors rely on medical tests and diagnostic tools (Gu, 1999). Given that TCM doctors are highly skilled communicators

(Wang, 2010), their approach fosters greater interpersonal communication between doctors and patients, providing more emotional support (Chung et al., 2009; Wang, 2010; Zhang & Sleeboom-Faulkner, 2011). Unlike WM, which targets symptom relief, TCM adopts a broader focus on both mental and physical health to identify the underlying imbalances that contribute to the symptoms.

Jin and Tay's (2017) comparative research on clinical interactions in WM and TCM consultations in mainland China revealed that TCM patients are more inclined to accept a comprehensive treatment plan for their entire body. Additionally, patients often believe their TCM practitioners have stronger communication skills than their WM counterparts (Wang, 2010), fostering long-term doctor-patient relationships and improving overall communication. Recently, there has been a growing focus on empowering patients and encouraging their participation in medical decision-making. This means patients are urged to express their treatment preferences and ask questions during consultations, allowing them to actively engage in diagnosis and treatment planning. Establishing effective communication between doctors and patients requires empowering patients to participate in decisions, which helps form the foundation for a positive therapeutic relationship and enhances adherence to treatment. In this collaborative approach, patients work alongside their doctors to manage their care. While recent studies have highlighted key aspects of TCM consultations, showing how the interactive methods of TCM practitioners help foster trust and strong therapeutic relationships, there remains a shortage of research examining the specifics of TCM consultations and how both doctors and patients interact collaboratively (Jin, 2018; Jin & Tay, 2017; Ho & Koenig, 2014). With this gap in mind, this study explored the distinct moments when TCM doctors use various physical examinations to assess patients' health conditions. Through discourse analysis, it was shown that TCM doctors provide both medical and emotional care, bridging the gap between their perspective on patient-centred care and that of their patients during crucial moments of physical examination.

Touch to understand

Observing through visual touches

As stated, the process of gathering information about a patient's health typically involves five key phases in TCM consultations, namely the four methods in si-zhen as well as maintaining contact and providing ongoing care. The first four stages work together to help both the practitioner and patient develop a shared understanding of the patient's health, allowing for more accurate diagnoses (Zheng et al., 2015). The initial phase, wang, involves practitioners observing physical symptoms to gather clues about underlying health issues (Pun et al., 2019). Practitioners examine various body parts such as the skin, hair, nails and tongue, as these can provide insights into the patient's overall condition. In excerpt 11.1, the use of wang as the initial diagnostic tool illustrates how practitioners assess patients' physical states through observation.

EXCERPT 11.1 (Notes: D = TCM practitioner, P1 = Patient 1)

12	D	好, 我幫你睇下吓。 = Ok, let me take a look for you. =
13	P1	= 好。 = OK.
14	D	OK。你呢:::條脷就係暗紅色嘅, 有啲脷苔。畀我睇下條脷。 OK. Your tongue is dark red in color, you have some fur on your tongue as well. Let me take a look at the tongue.
15	D	哦, 係喎。(0.1)裂痕。 Oh, yes. (0.1) a crack.
16	D	面色就係(0.1)偏黑啲, 面偏暗啲嘎, 嘴唇顏色正常嘅。 Your complexion looks a bit dark. But your lip colour is normal.
17	P1	係。 Yes.
18	D	噉脈象方面嚟講呢, 就係比較滑啲, 中醫嚟講嘎滑, 同埋(.)快啲。 Well, on the pulse, it rather slippery. Rather slippery, talking from TCM doctors' point of view. And it quite fast.
19	D	[體質。 [Constitution
20	P1	[滑係咩意思啊滑? [What does it mean by slippery?
21	D	滑呢, 就係痰濕比較重嘅。 = Slippery is, phlegmatic hygrosis. =
22	P1	= 嗯。 = uh-huh
23	D	痰濕比較重。 = Phlegmatic hygrosis =
24	P1	= 係, 冇錯。 = yes, that's right.
25	D	= 即係濕熱為主。 = = mainly, phlegmatic hygrosis =

Source: Adapted from Pun (2020).

As illustrated in lines 12–16, TCM practitioners usually begin by observing their patients' tongues, facial complexion and lip colour. In the consultation being discussed, the practitioner first noted that the patient's face appeared darker ('面色就係偏黑啲') and that their tongue had a crack and was dark red with some coating ('條脷就係暗紅色嘅, 有啲脷苔'). The TCM practitioner then mentioned that the patient's lip colour was normal ('嘴唇顏色正常嘅'). The patient acknowledged his own understanding of his condition in lines 17–25. From lines 14 to 16, the practitioner shared the results of his examination and his observations. In line 18, he offered insights into the patient's health based on these visible symptoms. To ensure the patient understood, the practitioner used everyday language like colloquial terms to explain the symptoms observed on different parts of the body, helping the patient grasp the medical concepts (Evans et al., 1986). By elaborating on his observations and providing a detailed account of the symptoms and diagnosis, the practitioner sought to reinforce the validity of his conclusions (Maynard & Heritage, 2005). At first, the patient struggled to grasp the diagnosis (Lines 18–20), but eventually, he understood his condition after the practitioner's use of simple, colloquial terms (Lines 21–23).

After briefly explaining his patient's condition, the practitioner continued to elaborate on his diagnosis in lines 23–25, noting that the patient's pulse was rapid. Based on his earlier observations of the patient's dark complexion and tongue, along with normal lip colour, he suggested the possibility of phlegmatic hygrosis affecting the patient's constitution. Initially, the patient was doubtful of this diagnosis. However, following the practitioner's clarification, the patient began to understand the meaning behind it. This case exemplifies how TCM practitioners use moments of 'touch' to achieve a shared understanding of health conditions by communicating through a common vocabulary (Evans et al., 1986). The excerpt illustrates how the practitioner combined 'visual touch' with the diagnostic process. By examining the patient's appearance, tongue and lip colour, the practitioner was able to interpret the health condition and offer possible explanations to aid the patient's understanding. Initially, when the practitioner used TCM-specific terms, the patient struggled to grasp them due to unfamiliarity. To bridge this gap, the practitioner provided a clearer explanation, emphasising the phlegmatic hygrosis in the patient's body. The patient eventually acknowledged the diagnosis and understood the practitioner's assessment.

Hear and smell to diagnose

After completing the wang stage, practitioners move on to the *wen* method, which involves listening and smelling to assess symptoms (Wang, 2010). In this phase, practitioners listen to their patients' coughs and the tone of their voices to evaluate their body constitutions. Additionally, they smell their patients' body odours and breath to gain insights into their health. Simultaneously, TCM practitioners consider their patients' medical histories and the effects of previous treatments from past consultations. By deepening their understanding of their patients' health backgrounds and experiences, practitioners can provide a more personalised diagnosis. However, in this particular study, the practitioner did not need to use the smelling aspect of *wen* during the recorded consultations, so the research team did not analyse that method.

EXCERPT 11.2 (Notes: D = TCM practitioner, P2 = Patient 2)

4	P2	誒我最主要呢就係(.)誒(0.1)即係而家講返好耐啦。 Erm my main problem is (.) er (0.1) it happened a long time ago.
5	D	嗯。 Okay.
6	P2	收經之前，收經之後呢。就係最主要呢就係(0.1)出汗同埋= Before menopause, after menopause. The main problem is(0.1)sweating and=
7	D	[收經之後 [after menopause
8	D	=倒汗? =night sweat?
9	P2	誒係喇。同埋係嗰個咩啊誒失眠好好緊要囉。 Yes. And I am having severe insomnia.
10	D	嗯嗯嗯。 Okay.
11	P2	噉我初期以為係(0.1)俎係一年呀至到五年啊咁。= I initially thought (0.1) it lasts one to five years=
12	D	[更年期呀。 [menopause?
13	D	= 就過喇。 = it will be over soon.
14	P2	但係我而家過咗咁多年呢我都(.)都冇乜改善。 But it doesn't improve over the years.
15	D	[都仍然有呢個情況。 [still have this situation.
16	P2	[係喇嘎。 [yes.
17	D	[明白。 [understood.

As for smelling, In the second excerpt from lines 4 to 14, the practitioner attentively listened as the patient described her menopause-related experiences.

She mentioned that she had been dealing with night sweats and insomnia since menopause began. Between lines 4 and 17, the practitioner allowed his patient time to share her experiences, indicating active listening. This encouraged her to provide essential details about her condition. The practitioner confirmed he was receiving her information by responding with 'Okay' and 'Understood' in lines 5 (嗯), 10 (嗯嗯嗯) and 17 (明白), showing his engagement with her comments. In lines 9–14, the patient asked for advice on addressing her night sweats and insomnia, indicating these issues had persisted for some time. By actively listening, the practitioner prompted her to share more about her situation, helping him gain a clearer understanding of her challenges. Thus, the excerpt illustrates how he utilised listening to achieve a deeper insight into his patient's condition, leading to more patient-centred evaluations and treatment plans. During the consultation, the practitioner created a moment of 'hearing touch' while diagnosing, focusing on the patients descriptions of her health history and concerns. He used conversational prompts like 'OK' in line 5 and inquired about symptoms such as 'night sweat?' in line 8, which the patient had overlooked. His responses indicated that he was attentive to her symptom description. He further confirmed his understanding by stating he 'understood in Line 17.

The importance of asking questions: Hidden details

The third phase of *si-zhen* is *wen*, which differs from the wen in the earlier stage. At this point, practitioners employ the method of *wen* to verbally inquire about their patients' conditions during consultations (Wang, 2010). By asking detailed questions, practitioners can gather information that may have been overlooked in the first two stages. They typically explore aspects that cannot be easily observed during the medical appointment, including dietary habits or bowel health. Since bowel conditions cannot be seen or smelt, it is crucial for practitioners to ask questions to gain a better understanding of the patient's overall health. During these sessions, practitioners clarify the significance of vital signs and primary symptoms concerning the patients' conditions. For example, in lines 19–30 in the third excerpt, the patient described his situation ambiguously several times. To gain clarity, the practitioner began to ask more specific questions such as 'How was the pain when you felt it?' in line 22 in order to better understand the pain and pinpoint the patient's main issue.

EXCERPT 11.3 (Notes: D = TCM practitioner, P3 = Patient 3)

19	D	即係停咗西藥之後呢(.)冇再感覺到好明顯嘅痛?= That is after discontinuing western medicine(.) Have you experience obvious pain again? =
20	P3	=誒:有嘅。即係亦都係扯(.)但係就冇強得好似佢佢初初一開始痛嘅時候咁咁痛嘍。起碼我可以姐係個頸擰覺得有啲痛嘅。 = um, yes. That is there is still gripping pain. But it wasn't as strong as when it first started. At least when I turn my head, it is just a bit painful.
21	D	[嗯:: [uh::
22	D	你嗰個嗰個痛即係你話果個突然之間:出嚟嗰個痛嘅時候係點樣樣?會唔會係都。 The pain you experienced, you mentioned it was a sudden pain. How was the pain when you felt it? Was it.
23	P3	[係呀。 [yes.
24	P3	=咪扯住囉。 = It was a gripping pain.
25	D	扯住我知。嗰個位置會唔會腫脹出嚟呀? I know it was gripping. But is that area swollen?
26	P3	唔覺得。我自己就摸唔倒佢佢佢腫脹。 I don't think so. I couldn't feel it swollen.
27	D	嗯。 Uh.
28	P3	=但就真係扯住痛。 = But the pain was really a gripping pain.
29	D	=嗯嗯。= = uh-huh =
30	P3	=[同埋今次呢((笑))就擘大個口食條粗啲嘅菜呢都痛啊。= = [also this time ((laugh)) I felt painful when I opened my mouth when eating a rather large piece of vegetable. =

The practitioner made additional efforts to follow up on the patient's report of muscle pain from lines 19 to 24. He inquired whether the patient experienced noticeable muscle discomfort after completing his Western medication in line 19 and also asked about the specific type of muscle pain in line 22. The patient described a gripping pain in his shoulder and neck region. By gathering this extra information through targeted questions, the practitioner gained a comprehensive understanding of the patient's muscle condition, enabling him to determine the most suitable and effective treatment for the pain.

To identify the potential causes of the muscle pain and provide more patient-centred care, the practitioner asked if there was any swelling in the affected area, as indicated in lines 25–26. He continued to follow up with additional questions regarding the pain and the specific painful area from lines 25 to 30. Throughout the interaction in lines 19–30, the patient emphasised his muscle discomfort, describing it as a gripping pain. The *wen* method enables practitioners to gain a thorough understanding of the patient's health and to comprehend their perceptions of discomfort, as well as the amount of effort they are willing to give to resolve the problem. This excerpt illustrates the practitioner's intent to provide patient-centred care, which fosters meaningful relationships between patients and practitioners. By listening, informing and involving his patient in self-care, the practitioner improved the consultation's effectiveness. According to Evans et al. (1986), doctors can significantly reduce the likelihood of overlooking potential ambiguities by employing questioning strategies that create a shared understanding of the symptoms. Consequently, this can reinforce patients' accurate perceptions of their issues. Thus, simply diagnosing is not enough; practitioners should ask questions about their patients' conditions to gather information that cannot be visually assessed.

Palpating: Physical touch as a means of identifying medical issues

TCM Practitioners utilise the *qie* method to touch and palpate various parts of the patient's body (Wang, 2010). By doing so, they can identify potential problems with muscles and joints, which is especially vital in orthopaedic assessments. Additionally, measuring the pulse allows practitioners to gain deeper insights into their patient's body constitutions. Through palpation or the act of feeling and measuring, they can assess the rhythm and strength of the heartbeat. Consequently, this technique aids them in understanding the patient's overall health and bodily conditions. It is standard practice for practitioners to check a patient's pulse and make health observations. Characteristics of the pulse such as depth, width and rhythm can indicate various symptoms related to both physical and mental health (Tang et al., 2012). For example, a slippery and wide pulse may suggest issues like food stagnation in the intestines or phlegmatic hygrosis.

EXCERPT 11.4 (Notes: D = TCM practitioner, P4 = Patient 4)

Except 4. D = TCM practitioner, P4 = Patient 4

18	D	噉脈象方面嚟講呢，就係比較滑喲，中醫嚟講嘎滑，同埋(.)快喲。 Well, on the pulse, it's rather slippery. Rather slippery, talking from TCM doctors' point of view. And it quite fast.
19	D	[體質。 [Constitution.
20	P4	[滑係咩意思啊滑? [What does it mean by slippery?
21	D	滑呢，就係痰濕比較重嘅。 = Slippery is, phlegmatic hygrosis. =
22	P4	=嗯。 =uh-huh.
23	D	痰濕比較重。 = Phlegmatic hygrosis =
24	P4	=係，冇錯。 =yes, that's right.
25	D	數啊，即係數學個數啦，噉數啊快。 = math, that is mathematics, so its fast. =
26	P4	=係係。 =yes yes.

27	D	=即係濕熱為主。= =mainly, phlegmatic hygrosis =
28	P4	=嗯= =uh=
29	D	=嗯。 =uh-huh.
30	D	噉呢頭先分析出嚟你個體質呢，係濕熱為主嘅。 So we just analysed your constitution, which is mainly phlegmatic hygrosis
31	P4	嗯嗯嗯。 Uh-huh.
32	D	兼有氣虛同埋陰虛。(0.2)就係噉喇。 Also your qi and yin are weak. (0.2) that's that.

In a recorded consultation shown in the fourth excerpt, lines 18–27 (see arrow) noted the practitioner starting to measure the patient's pulse and discuss his findings. He identified a slippery pulse, indicating phlegmatic hygrosis in the patient's body constitution, and also noted that the pulse was relatively fast. Bouhdili (2015) pointed out that pulse qualities such as width, strength and rate reflect different bodily conditions. The practitioner observed that the patient's pulse was both slippery and fast, which suggested an excess of head and phlegm accumulation, consistent with symptoms of phlegmatic hygrosis. TCM practitioners often use the term 'body constitution' to describe the balance or imbalance within bodily systems (Al-Shura, 2014). Factors such as the environment, emotions, spirituality and medical conditions can influence this constitution. After measuring the pulse and making initial observations, the practitioner stated that the patient exhibited *qi* and *yin* deficiency in line 32, indicated by the weak pulse (Wu et al., 2013). He mentioned that the patient might be experiencing fatigue, insomnia, low blood pressure or depression simultaneously.

At first, the patient struggled to grasp the meaning of *qi* and *yin* deficiency. Therefore, from lines 18 to 30, the practitioner elaborated on his observations regarding the patient's pulse and his diagnosis. With this detailed explanation, the patient was able to understand the practitioner's comments and agreed with the assessment. In TCM, palpation is a crucial technique as it serves as a primary method for the evaluation of health in major organ systems and mental states (Zheng et al., 2015). In this instance, the practitioner highlighted three characteristics of the patient's pulse: fast, weak and slippery. These observations suggested that the patient had concerns related to excess heat, fatigue and phlegmatic hygrosis within their body constitution.

Making a connection: Being in touch for long-term practitioner-patient relationships

In the consultations analysed, the practitioner initiated discussions with his patients using a socio-relational approach. He engaged in small talk such as greetings and farewells (Jin, 2018), which helped establish a connection and foster a friendly environment. This approach facilitated the development of trusting relationships between the practitioner and his patients. By demonstrating empathy and building rapport, the practitioner was better able to understand his patients' health conditions and provide patient-centred diagnoses (Slade et al., 2015a; 2015b).

EXCERPT 11.5 (Notes: D = TCM practitioner, P5 = Patient 5)

1	D	好(.)嗯(.)呢排點樣先?= Ok, uh, how are you recently?=
2	P5	=誒:誒:= =um, um=
3	D	=個情況。 =the situation.
4	P5	都:係差唔多, 但好容易攰呢排。 Well, pretty much the same, but I easily get tired recently.
5	D	好容易攰?= Easily tired?=
6	P5	=係喇。 =yeah.
7	D	點解?你唔係話完成曬啲(.)學校啲野咩? Why? Didn't you say you're finished with school stuff?
8	P5	哦唔係吖, 跟住完成曬嗰啲要務之後= Oh no, after finishing those =
9	D	=((笑))又做咩?= =((laugh))what now?=
10	P5	=誒(.)就誒啱啱::尋日就係最後一日返學。 = =ugh,(.)just now::yesterday was the last day of school. =
11	D	=[係。 =[yes
12	P5	[咁又有好多啲畢業禮啊= [there are many graduation ceremonies. =
13	D	=[畢業禮哦 =[graduation ceremonies

As demonstrated in the conversation captured between lines 7 and 13, the practitioner seldom addressed his patient's health issues directly. For instance, he inquired, 'Didn't you say you're finished with school stuff?' in line 7. The question concerned more with the patient's lifestyle than any biomedical topic. This indicated the practitioner's effort to create a friendly environment by engaging with the patient about her schedule. In line 9, he asked, 'What now?' to show empathy towards her busy lifestyle, indicating his understanding of her situation. The patient's response suggested her willingness to cultivate a positive and friendly atmosphere with the practitioner. By maintaining a warm demeanour, the practitioner strengthened the practitioner-patient relationship. Thus, TCM practitioners utilise small talk to foster connections with patients. Relying solely on palpation is insufficient for gathering all necessary information. To identify pulse imbalances, practitioners must ask more socio-relational questions (Jin, 2018). Overall, employing the five types of 'touches' outlined in the results section can enhance the effectiveness of consultations between practitioners and their patients.

A summary of the communication flow in TCM consultations

TCM practice is recognised for providing a comprehensive understanding of patients' needs in physical, psychological and emotional dimensions, emphasising a patient-centred approach in care and services. Studies revealed several interactional stages during consultations that enable practitioners to progressively move from assessing patients' health conditions to achieving a mutual understanding through various forms of 'touches' (See more from Pun, 2020). After these 'touches', patients grasp their practitioners' explanations and interpret the implications of their diagnoses or deficiencies in their body constitutions. The types of 'touches' include visual, auditory/olfactory, verbal, physical and maintaining connection. These interactions help practitioners understand both the medical and social factors influencing their patients' health holistically. By gaining insights into their patients' daily habits, emotions and behaviours, practitioners can create more effective treatment plans that support overall balance. The excerpts in the findings highlight the importance of small talk, as it encourages patients to participate and engage more actively in their care. Figure 3.1 summarises the communication flow.

Traditional Chinese Medicine (TCM) consultations follow a structured yet dynamic communication flow that enables practitioners to gain a holistic understanding of patients' physical, psychological and emotional well-being. Rooted in a patient-centred approach, TCM practice emphasises deep engagement through various interactional stages. This study identifies five key stages of interaction – *Observation (Visual Touch)*, *Auscultation/Olfaction (Hearing/Smelling)*, *Inquiry (Verbal Touch)*, *Palpation (Physical Touch)* and *Maintaining Connection (Staying in Touch)* – which progressively guide both the practitioner and patient towards a mutual understanding of the patient's health condition and treatment plan.

Each stage of communication plays a crucial role in diagnosing and treating patients while fostering a trusting doctor-patient relationship. Through these stages, practitioners not only assess symptoms but also engage in meaning-making processes that allow patients to comprehend and internalise the implications of their diagnoses and body constitutions.

1. *Observation (Visual Touch)*

   The consultation begins with the TCM practitioner visually examining the patient's appearance, including their complexion, posture and other external signs that might indicate underlying health issues. The practitioner describes these observations and provides preliminary interpretations using TCM terminology. Given that some patients may not be familiar with these terms, they often seek clarification. The practitioner then adapts their explanations into more colloquial expressions to ensure comprehension. This process allows patients to actively engage in the consultation, ask questions and gradually build their understanding of their health conditions.
2. *Auscultation/Olfaction (Hearing/Smelling)*

   In this stage, the patient is encouraged to share their daily habits, lifestyle and personal experiences related to their health concerns. The TCM practitioner assumes an active listening role, prompting the patient to disclose relevant health information. During this dialogue, the practitioner may suggest other possible but related symptoms for the patient to consider. The patient may either affirm or challenge these suggestions, which further refines the diagnostic process. By integrating patient narratives with their clinical knowledge, the practitioner formulates a patient-centred diagnosis and tailors treatment recommendations accordingly. This stage reinforces trust and helps identify hidden health issues that the patient may not have initially recognised.
3. *Inquiry (Verbal Touch)*

   Building on the previous stages, the practitioner asks targeted questions to explore additional aspects of the patient's health that may not have been spontaneously mentioned. The patient describes their bodily sensations, symptoms and overall condition. The practitioner then poses follow-up questions to refine the diagnosis, often suggesting other symptoms that the patient might not have considered relevant. This exchange allows for a deeper understanding of the patient's condition and helps bridge potential gaps between clinical observations and patient experiences. At the conclusion of this stage, the practitioner formulates a diagnostic judgement using TCM principles and terminology, further advancing the collaborative nature of the consultation.

4. *Palpation (Physical Touch)*

   At this stage, the TCM practitioner conducts pulse diagnosis, a fundamental technique in TCM used to assess the balance of *qi*, blood flow and organ function. The practitioner first describes their findings and provides an initial diagnosis. Patients may seek additional explanations, prompting the practitioner to use more accessible language to facilitate understanding. The physical interaction in this stage serves not only as a diagnostic tool but also as a means to reassure patients. As a result, patients often express agreement with the diagnosis and demonstrate increased confidence in the treatment plan.

5. *Maintaining Connection (Staying in Touch)*

   To conclude the consultation, the practitioner engages in small talk, fostering a relaxed and open communication environment. This stage helps strengthen the doctor-patient relationship by encouraging patients to share more about their daily routines, emotions and lifestyle choices. If the patient is initially reserved, the practitioner may ask specific but non-intrusive questions to encourage further discussion. Through this exchange, the practitioner gathers additional contextual information that may inform future treatment adjustments. The consultation ends with the practitioner expressing empathy and understanding, reinforcing the patient's sense of care and support.

The structured yet flexible communication flow in TCM consultations highlights the intricate interplay between medical expertise and interpersonal rapport. By employing multiple forms of 'touches' – visual, auditory, verbal and physical – practitioners create a multidimensional diagnostic process that transcends mere symptom analysis. This approach allows for a holistic integration of medical, psychological and social factors, enabling a personalised and patient-centred treatment plan.

Additionally, the progressive nature of the communication stages ensures that patients play an active role in the consultation, gradually developing a deeper understanding of their health conditions. The use of colloquial explanations, active listening and interactive questioning bridges the gap between medical knowledge and patient comprehension, enhancing treatment adherence and patient satisfaction.

Finally, maintaining an ongoing connection beyond the diagnostic process reinforces trust and long-term engagement, which is particularly important in TCM's emphasis on balance and preventive care. By fostering open and empathetic communication, TCM practitioners encourage sustained patient involvement in their health management, ultimately improving health outcomes.

This refined understanding of TCM consultation dynamics provides valuable insights for enhancing communication training among practitioners and optimising patient-practitioner interactions.

Learning from TCM's metaphorical and physical touches: Insights for non-Asian doctors to show empathy and give support

The act of touching involves lightly placing our hands or other body parts onto something or someone (Cambridge Dictionary, 2019). Within the realm of TCM practice, touch plays a crucial role in patient-centred care as it allows practitioners to thoroughly assess their patients' health conditions and senses, thus leading to more holistic diagnoses and treatment plans. Rooted in the principle of holism, TCM considers everything interconnected (Wu et al., 2013). Illnesses are perceived as manifestations of specific deficiencies in a patient's body. TCM treatment may involve various strategies, such as increased rest, dietary changes and mood adjustments, alongside acupuncture and herbal remedies. Additionally, small talk in TCM consultations serves to create an environment where patients can discuss their lifestyles, emotions and dietary habits in addition to the biomedical aspects of their conditions (Jin, 2018).

Furthermore, practitioners should physically assess their patients' pulses, observe their tongues and smell their breath (Pun, 2020). In TCM, the term 'touch' is often used metaphorically to illustrate the nature of interactions within the practice. Practitioners typically use the four methods of *si-zhen* for diagnosis (Zheng et al., 2015). According to Gu (1999), these personalised 'touches' embody the wisdom inherent in TCM philosophy, which contrasts with WM. In WM, physicians rely on laboratory diagnostics and instruments, which reduces personal involvement and minimises bias. While WM primarily targets symptoms, TCM focuses on treating the individual.

The research team observed that TCM practitioners use the term 'touch' differently, particularly in relation to pulse diagnosis, unlike WM doctors who measure heart rates primarily for blood pressure monitoring during standard physical exams. In TCM, pulse diagnosis is regarded as a sophisticated art, requiring trained practitioners to perform evaluations through touch. By applying a gentle touch to a patient's arm, practitioners can discern up to twenty-eight different pulse qualities, such as rate, strength and width. For example, a rapid pulse may indicate excessive 'heat' in the body, whereas a slow pulse suggests a 'cold' condition that hinders bodily function. On top of that, a strong pulse may reflect an excess of certain elements, indicating stress or high blood pressure, while many elderly patients exhibit a weak pulse, signifying deficiencies that could lead to fatigue or low blood pressure. A slippery pulse might indicate digestive issues, such as food stagnation or phlegm buildup. These pulse qualities allow practitioners to pinpoint specific health issues and locations within the body. Therefore, these 'touches' provide essential insights into patients' health, facilitating physical assessments of internal conditions. The pulse serves as a valuable tool for both practitioners and patients, fostering a deeper understanding of the connections between body, mind and lifestyle. Thus, 'touches' are vital in the diagnostic process during TCM consultations, enabling biomedical discussions.

These 'touches' also offer interactive support, as Chinese medicine creates a platform for various communication styles among practitioners. Each of the five types of 'touches' represents a distinct communication dynamic between practitioners and patients (see Figure 3.1). Consultations should be maintained as two-way interactions (Jin, 2018; Jin & Tay, 2017) as effective two-way communication is crucial for providing patient-centred care (Slade et al., 2015a; 2015b; Ribeiro & Hoyle, 2009). For instance, while practitioners initiate conversations, patients tend to contribute significantly. During the hearing/smelling touches, patients share their experiences, symptoms and feelings, while practitioners primarily listen and analyse the information conveyed through verbal communication. TCM practitioners are expected to practise active listening, respond appropriately and show empathy. Additionally, practitioners should be skilled at questioning to gather information that is not visually apparent during verbal touches. At this stage, it is important for

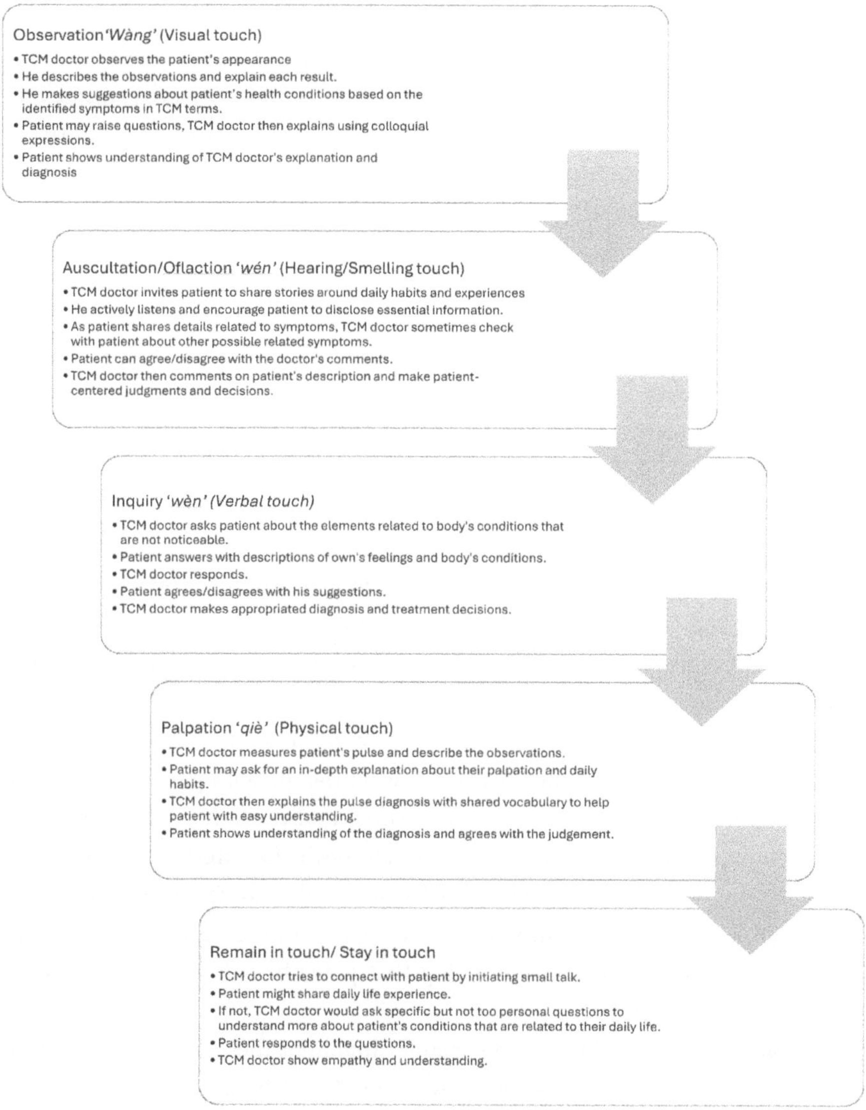

Figure 3.1 Traditional Chinese Medicine communication flow in action

practitioners to be careful and strategic when posing questions, ensuring they are both informative and personal (Jin & Tay, 2017). The same applies to the last type of 'touch', which involves maintaining contact. While small talk can foster engagement and friendly relationships, it risks becoming intrusive or inappropriate if practitioners lack strong communication skills. Thus, TCM practitioners must develop excellent communication abilities. Although this study focused on specific ideal communication patterns through a convenient sample, it provides valuable insights for future researchers and TCM educators, facilitating the creation of more comprehensive training programmes in doctor-patient communication. Future research should explore additional communication interventions used by TCM practitioners during consultations to enhance patient-centred approaches in diverse contexts.

*

While WM prioritises symptom management, TCM focuses on facilitating healing for patients. Engaging in small talk is especially significant because it helps practitioners gather more insights regarding their patients' physical conditions and social circumstances, enabling TCM professionals to create more comprehensive treatment plans. Evans et al. (1986) emphasise the importance of establishing a mutual understanding between practitioners and patients as a foundation for diagnosis and treatment. Therefore, the role of TCM practitioners extends beyond identifying the causes of patients' issues. It also involves exploring the conceptual framework that fosters a shared understanding of these concerns. When practitioners and patients have differing perspectives on issues, it can lead to inaccurate diagnoses and treatment noncompliance, resulting in unsuccessful medical outcomes. Thus, it is essential for both parties to cultivate a mutual understanding of the patient's health conditions through the practice of 'touching', which reflects a cultural approach to internalising illnesses by addressing problems within the patients' bodily systems. Findings that concerned TCM communication could be applied to the designs of culturally appropriate insights into WM, ensuring that patients' cultural and emotional needs are well-catered to.

To conclude, the findings in this chapter highlight the intricate and holistic communication strategies employed by Traditional Chinese Medicine (TCM) practitioners to foster meaningful interactions with their patients. Through the integration of multiple forms of 'touch' – visual, auditory, verbal and physical – TCM consultations go beyond mere symptom analysis to construct a patient-centred approach that values the interconnectedness of physical, psychological and social well-being. The study underscores how TCM communication effectively builds trust, encourages patient engagement and supports shared decision-making. Additionally, the long-term practitioner-patient relationships cultivated in TCM contrast with the often transactional nature of Western medical consultations, reinforcing the significance of continuity and cultural sensitivity in healthcare.

The insights gained from TCM communication are not only valuable within the realm of traditional medicine but also offer broader implications for other medical contexts, particularly in end-of-life (EOL) communication. As we transition to the next chapter, we shift our focus to oncology and palliative care, examining how cultural beliefs, communication barriers and family dynamics influence EOL discussions in Chinese contexts. By exploring the challenges and strategies of delivering difficult news and navigating familial expectations, Chapter 4 will build upon the communication themes established in TCM practice, providing further understanding of how medical discourse shapes patient care and decision-making at critical stages of life.

4

Oncology and palliative care

Why is End-Of-Life (EOL) communication in Chinese contexts ineffective?

End-Of-Life (EOL) conversations offer dying patients and healthcare providers a chance to talk about treatment expectations and what future issues the patients may face (Pun et al., 2020). These conversations are beneficial to both parties and the caregivers (Wright et al., 2008). Previous research has demonstrated that patients who have high involvement in EOL discussions often receive less aggressive medical care and thus have a higher quality of life at the end of their life, and their caregivers are also less likely to experience depression (Epstein & Street, 2007). Moreover, by encouraging discussions between dying patients and healthcare professionals, clinicians can achieve more desirable treatment outcomes with lower medical costs, based on a mutual agreement on budgets and expectations towards treatments (Zhang et al., 2009).

That being said, it is challenging for clinicians to initiate EOL discussions with their patients as a lot of oncologists and nurses find it difficult, or have not tried to, to put themselves in their patients' shoes when delivering bad news (Fan et al., 2019). While it is only understandable that medical professionals want to be more empathetic during EOL conversations, it is also necessary for them to understand that their patients would expect a balance between factual and emotional help (Hack et al., 2005). To be specific, it is essential for clinicians to address and acknowledge patients' emotional responses and feelings on top of the actual medical treatment, which prevents their patients from feeling abandoned (Dias et al., 2003). In order to close the gap between fulfilling patients' medical and interpersonal needs in EOL communication, many studies have introduced protocols and approaches to help medical professionals deliver bad news (Pun et al., 2020). For example, Villagran et al.'s (2010) 'COMFORT' (Communication, Orientation, Mindfulness, Family, Ongoing, Reiterative messages and Team) model illustrates a set of principles aimed at offering a step-by-step guide on how to deliver unsettling news while offering comfort and being humane in such conversations. Another common six-step protocol, 'SPIKES' (Setting, Perception, Invitation, Knowledge, Empathetic Response, Summary), also aids doctors in preparing properly for delivering bad news to their patients (Schpira, 2006).

Unfortunately, these established communicative models might be validated in most non-Asian settings and thus are not suitable for Chinese EOL communication contexts. This is due to the fact that patients from different cultural backgrounds have different communicative needs (Pun et al., 2020). Chinese people and medical professionals have different beliefs and practices in terms of EOL care when compared to those of the English-speaking world. Clinicians often hesitate to disclose prognoses to terminally ill patients due to cultural perspectives on a 'good death', which is considered a taboo subject in Chinese philosophy (Pun et al., 2020). A number of research projects have demonstrated that prevailing Chinese cultural influences lead to the negligence of the need for effective communication about terminal illnesses in relevant settings. Therefore, it is inappropriate for clinicians in Chinese societies, oncologists and palliative care providers, in particular, to directly employ Western models in EOL discussions. A culturally appropriate framework for EOL care should be developed to fit the needs of Chinese patients.

This chapter addresses this need by reviewing previous studies that have explored EOL communication between oncologists, palliative care providers and their patients in a range of Chinese settings, highlighting certain cultural influences, suggesting communication strategies for EOL conversations, and the implications of TCM communication styles on EOL care.

Factors that define the nature of EOL communication in Chinese contexts: The underlying Confucian, Taoist and Buddhist philosophies behind the concept of a 'good death'

Influenced greatly by various Chinese philosophies, Chinese societies have formed their own unique perspectives on dying and death in the past four millennia (Cui et al., 2011; Hsu et al., 2009; Wang et al., 2004; Zheng et al., 2015), which are distinctive from that of the Western countries. The concept of 'good death' has been developed on the basis of Confucianism, Taoism and Buddhism (Chan et al., 2006). Such a concept has generated direct implications for clinical practices, particularly in terms of the communication style of EOL conversations with dying patients and their bereaved families (Pun et al., 2020). In a project conducted in Hong Kong, Mak (2001) identified seven elements of a good death, including (1) the awareness of dying, (2) maintaining a sense of hope, (3) being pain-free and not suffering, (4) having control over one's EOL experience, (5) getting prepared to depart and (6) being able to accept the timing of one's decease.

The above seven elements imply that accepting death in Chinese societies is a shared decision that is determined by one's social role in a family, instead of a personal choice (Pun et al., 2020). Hsu et al.'s (2009) study demonstrated that good death is not shaped by one's actual age but by one's ability to fulfil familial responsibilities. Old age indirectly suggests good death as older patients are seen as more likely to have fulfilled their familial roles and be able to accept when they could do no work for the family (Hsu et al., 2009). In another study conducted in Hong Kong by Chan (2011), fifteen bereaved Chinese elderly women aged between 66 and 86 years, whose husbands had deceased 8.5 to 62 months prior shared in interviews that the elements of a good death that they had wished for their late husbands were similar to those observed in former studies, including minimal suffering in EOL, presence of the family when dying, harmonious family relationships, natural death and not being a burden to other people.

While we have approached the twenty-first century, negative attitudes towards EOL discussions are still prevalent in Chinese societies (Zheng et al., 2015; Wong-Kim et al., 2003). When forming EOL care plans, a lot of Chinese patients are affected by Chinese philosophies and find advance-care planning disruptive to their emotional balance as they focus on negative thoughts (Bowman & Singer, 2003). The majority of Chinese people, including clinicians, are often unwilling to talk about death for fear of bringing bad luck (Wang et al., 2004; Tse et al., 2003). To be specific, some Chinese elderly people are superstitious and think that discussing death implies bad luck and that the discussion will 'invite' death to approach sooner (Chi et al., 2018; Yonashiro-Cho et al., 2016). Such cultural taboos make it challenging for clinicians and families to begin EOL conversations, considering that elderly people are quite sensitive to subjects regarding death.

A lot of Chinese patients and their family members are reluctant to be informed of a terminal diagnosis (Zhang & Liu, 2010). Therefore, a lot of cancer patients are prevented from being told of their declining health conditions, even when they have reached the terminal stage (Pun et al., 2020). Such a cultural issue makes it difficult for clinicians to disclose information to Chinese cancer patients. This part of communication has been deemed the most difficult for healthcare workers, even for nursing staff who communicate with terminal patients the most (Dong & Yin, 2012).

Chinese patients who have a more comprehensive grasp of their conditions, a more advanced level of education or higher Western acculturation tend to be more open to the thought of planning their own EOL matters (Pun et al., 2020). According to Ko and Lee's (2009) study, patients with better knowledge regarding advance-care planning usually participate more in EOL conversations.

It is a taboo: Does talking about death really bring bad luck?

In a lot of Chinese traditions, talking about death is seen as a cultural taboo (Yanoshiro-Cho et al., 2016; Fielding & Hung, 1996; Fielding et al., 1994). As stated, many Chinese elderly people always refuse to make advance directives due to their belief of talking about death brings bad luck (Pun et al., 2020). Without the presence of an actual condition, advance-care planning might appear to be quite abstract and rather hypothetical. However, a lot of older patients are open to the idea of considering advance directives when they are actually suffering from serious illnesses, including disclosure of terminal diagnoses and prognoses (Tse et al., 2003; Ko et al., 2003). Clinicians can keep track of the ability and willingness of their patients to determine the best time to start a conversation about advance-care planning with their patients as well as their families.

Medicine is considered a highly regarded profession in Chinese societies. As a result, patients have a lot of respect for their doctors and depend on their clinicians for medical information and details about their diagnoses. Chinese patients tend to have high expectations for their doctors: clinicians are expected to offer a comprehensive overview of their diagnoses and other additional information that may help them in managing and making EOL decisions (Fan et al., 2019). It is crucial for practitioners to elaborate on all available options complemented with an appropriate amount of scientific information to offer their patients an all-round picture of their illnesses and prognoses, and then guide them to make satisfactory EOL decisions (Fielding & Hung, 1996).

In Chinese medical contexts, a power differential between doctors and their patients is often observed (Wang, 2010). In Mainland China, in particular, doctors often play the authorial role while their patients are rather passive. In these contexts, patients are often expected to talk less and mostly listen to their doctors without raising many questions. Otherwise, they may be deemed challenging their doctors' authority (Pun et al., 2020). However, the roles and social status of practitioners and their patients have evolved in the past few decades and become more and more balanced. Therefore, both patients and clinicians have to develop trust to carry out open conversations.

Another extremely important feature of the Chinese perspective on EOL conversations is the collectivist family-centred attitude (Sun et al., 2011). While a lot of people think that terminally ill patients have the right to learn about their diagnoses and the stage of their physical conditions, a huge number of Chinese families refuse to let the doctors inform their elderly family members of such factual information (Zheng et al., 2015; Wong-Kim et al., 2003). The collectivist nature of Chinese cultural values contrasts starkly with the individualist values advocated in the West. Chinese patients mostly prefer discussing matters with their families before making a shared decision (Pun et al., 2020). In Chinese societies, a lot of elderly patients let their children make EOL decisions on their behalf as they think their offspring have a good understanding of their preferences (Fan et al., 2019; Tse et al., 2003; Fielding & Hung, 1996).

When dealing with EOL care in Chinese medical settings, nurses tend to focus on their terminally ill patients' physical comfort and wish fulfilment. On the other hand, doctors emphasise their patients' rights as well as symptom management (Chan et al., 2006). However, their approaches are not ideal as the voice of patients hoping to learn more about their conditions is highly neglected due to the intense predilection of family-centred traditions (Pun et al., 2020). According to Tang et al.'s (2006) study in Taiwan, there were substantial discrepancies between terminally ill patients and their families regarding the extent to which they were told about their diagnoses and prognoses. Tang et al.'s (2006) data illustrated a contradiction of terminally ill patients' expectations, who, despite the influences of collectivist values, stressed their absolute right to be informed directly by their clinicians over their families. Therefore, doctors are required to respect their patients' preferences instead of just routinely prioritising the families' opinions when a disagreement arises.

It is often stressful and quite demanding for clinicians to communicate EOL matters with their patients and their families. Chinese clinicians adopt a passive approach to disclosing prognoses. Just as I discussed earlier on, the Chinese cultural preference for avoiding bad news delivery has a key role in this process, as proven by a study of palliative care providers in China (Chan et al., 2006). The interviewees in this study said that they were requested by their patients' families not to inform the patients of their health conditions. As a result, effective communication was prevented between clinicians and their dying patients, putting emotional support at risk and leading to clinicians' moral distress and frustration (Chan et al., 2006).

In Zheng et al.'s (2015) study, oncologists described caring for their patients' negative emotions as the most challenging part of their job. Nurses who worked in palliative care also noted that they did not have adequate knowledge of their patients' psychological needs, making it urgent for them to learn more about the psycho-social changes experienced by their patients in the EOL stage (Chan et al., 2006). There is an obvious need for medical educators to train Chinese nurses as many in Hsu et al.'s (2009) study ranked 'communication with dying patients' the second most important in their learning priorities for EOL training, two rankings higher than 'physical care of dying patients'.

Communicative strategies for oncologists

One of the key research topics is the design of communication strategies for oncologists to break bad news in EOL conversations (Pun et al., 2020). The model of patient-centred care has turned into the most preferred approach for medical professionals to offer quality palliative care. On the other hand, provider-oriented goals are also useful in shaping what healthcare professionals say and offer insights into the ideal medical outcome of EOL discussions. While the latter communication style is not encouraged in most EOL discussions, it can nevertheless be integrated into part of the healthcare plans to aid clinicians in achieving clinicians' desired outcomes for their dying patients (Russell, 2016). A study revealed that when breaking bad news, clinicians usually lack a specific goal, or do not consider how such news may influence the receivers or if anyone should be with the patients when they receive such shocking news (Ptacek et al., 1999). Clinicians usually face difficulties when relaying information regarding terminal illnesses. Such challenges tend to impair the progress of medical consultations, and it is significant to understand these challenges in order to help clinicians overcome them (Dias et al., 2003). However, it is impossible to design a formulaic approach as EOL conversations should be tailored to patients' perspectives, the contexts and the content of the conversations (Sparks et al., 2007).

Other factors that influence EOL conversations are cultural competence and familial influences (Pun et al., 2020). Medical professionals are required to consider their patients' perspectives and be attentive to and respect their cultural values, which allows them to develop a trusting and collaborative relationship with their dying patients (Barclay et al., 2007). Gaining approval and support from patients' families can reassure the clinicians that the patients' values are respected, which also stabilises and strengthens their familial bonds (Scott & Caughlin, 2014). The following section outlines key communication strategies that clinicians can employ to enhance end-of-life (EOL) discussions with patients and their families in Asian contexts. By incorporating culturally sensitive approaches, healthcare professionals can foster trust, improve patient comprehension and facilitate shared decision-making, ultimately ensuring a more patient-centred and compassionate EOL experience. These strategies include indirect communication, involving family members in decision-making, initiating EOL discussions at the right time, tailoring difficult conversations, promoting health literacy, increasing cultural awareness, implementing patient-centred care, encouraging patient communication, recognising the role of nurses and adopting questioning techniques from Traditional Chinese Medicine (TCM) to foster deeper engagement.

1) *Indirect communication*

   Former studies have proven that indirect communication is greatly encouraged by Asian patients in EOL discussions. There are specific tactics for clinicians to initiate EOL discussions to make sure that the conversations will be comfortable for the patients (Pun et al., 2021b). For example, clinicians are encouraged to use non-verbal cues and body language to gauge a discussion. The tone of voice, manner and attitude are also important in terms of gauging patients' willingness to be involved in EOL conversation (Bezemer et al., 2017). Indirect communication minimises the pressure brought by face-to-face verbal interactions and offers the patients a chance to decline the discussions non-verbally (Kwak & Salmon, 2007; Bowman & Singer, 2001; Chi et al., 2018). Other effective approaches include depersonalising the conversations by framing them as standard questions by policy and using other EOL care experiences as illustrated examples (Im et al., 2019).
2) *Considering families' opinions in a collectivist context*

   Being able to recognise the role of family in EOL conversations is a useful skill for oncologists. Former studies have demonstrated that family members often play an important role in different stages including diagnosis, receiving shocking news, making shared decisions on treatment plans and planning palliate care (Scott, 2010; Keeley, 2016; McDarby et al., 2019). Oncologists should understand the importance and influence of patients' families and learn how to involve them in EOL conversations as well as utilise their influence to their patients' benefit. Oncologists should be trained to identify hidden agendas including family dynamics and strive to consider the caregivers' perspectives as a crucial source during decision-making processes because they have a good understanding of the patients' preferences and are critical to effective communication and desirable outcomes (Abbey, 2008).

3) *Initiating EOL conversations timely*

It is necessary for oncologists to learn when to initiate EOL discussions with their dying patients and their family caregivers (Pun et al., 2021). It is not unusual for terminally ill patients to be hesitant to involve in EOL discussions, and it can greatly affect their quality of life as well as treatment decisions. A lot of Chinese patients prefer not to be told about their diagnoses and delay their EOL decisions to deny the reality of their conditions (Fielding & Hung, 1996; Im et al., 2019). Oncologists should initiate EOL discussions with their dying patients as soon as possible. By doing so, the patients can gain a simple overview of palliative care and advance directives, so they can accept and begin advanced care planning (Pun et al., 2021).

4) *Tailoring difficult conversations: informing patients of the natural course of illnesses in various stages*

It is significant for oncologists to mentally prepare their patients for a long and continual EOL process. Oncologists have to learn how to carry out EOL conversations with these patients during various stages of illnesses, which include times when the patients feel well during medical treatments when admissions turn into more frequent visits and patients become weaker, and when they actually reach the stage in which they are approaching their deaths.

5) *Promoting health literacy using standardised content coverage*

Oncologists are required to cover a number of topics, including disclosing their patients' current status and prognoses to discuss their illnesses with data and information (Pun et al., 2021). By using relevant information and figures, their patients can better understand their own health conditions and make the most suitable EOL decisions. It is particularly crucial for oncologists in Asia to lay out all possible options for their patients as doctors are considered authorial figures and the main source of medical information on illnesses and treatment options, whom patients have a lot of trust in (Abbey, 2008; Wang, 2010; Pun et al., 2018). In order to advocate better health literacy and self-management skills and give oneself more confidence, oncologists are encouraged to give their patients a preview of the future symptoms and changes in accordance with one's particular symptoms. Eventually, oncologists should elaborate on future care needs and options and attempt to understand their patients' preferences. They should explain choices regarding palliative and EOL care like resuscitation, institutionalisation, or home treatments to their patients, so the patients can make informed decisions when the time arrives. On top of that, addressing patients' particular concerns can minimise their psychological stress and aid them in creating a better experience in the EOL stage. It is important for oncologists to correct any misunderstandings regarding their respective illnesses and talk about how to communicate with families. Former studies have proven that families can generate a positive influence on patients during EOL conversations as they can offer emotional support and physical care (Odgers et al., 2018).

6) *Increasing cultural awareness*

Being culturally aware of cultural elements that shape EOL contexts is a key factor in forming a comfortable and satisfying EOL experience for terminally ill patients. Each culture has its own concept of dying based on religions, traditions and beliefs (Jin, 2018). While it is impossible for oncologists to be knowledgeable about all cultures, they should acquire cultural knowledge about the community they are usually treating and try to learn about the philosophies behind EOL conversations. Being culturally competent allows oncologists to facilitate effective EOL communication and make the conversations easier for patients as they reach the end of their life (Pun et al., 2021).

7) *Implementing patient-centred care and understanding the power dynamics between healthcare professionals and patients*

While there is a typical power dynamic in Chinese societies in which patients are expected to play the passive role and not challenge their doctors' authority (McDarby et al., 2019), oncologists should still understand that the approach of patient-centred care is typically recommended for clinical communication (Pun et al., 2021). By implementing patient-centred communication during EOL discussions, patients can experience a better quality of holistic medical care (Jin, 2018; Im et al., 2019). To carry out patient-centred care, oncologists should (1) be attentive to their patients' needs, be mindful of their personal experiences and thoughts and (2) invite them to be part of their recovery processes, thus improving doctor-patient relationships (Epstein & Street, 2007).

8) *Encouraging patients to communicate their needs and forming trusting relationships*

   By making suggestions about skills on how to deliver bad news to their ill family members, oncologists can guide patients' families to ease their relatives' minds and offer support to build trusting relationships (Pun et al., 2021). As stated, while communication strategies like non-verbal language can be used in both Asian and Western EOL contexts, it is essential for oncologists to tailor to Asian patients' needs in order to express care and be empathetic (Pun et al., 2021). Asian patients' needs are always unfulfilled. Therefore, clinicians need to be trained to use culturally specific communication strategies for EOL discussions.

9) *The role of nurses: guiding patients and families to make EOL decisions*

   The participation of family caregivers during the early stage of EOL communication can make sure that patients' EOL decisions can be efficiently executed (Pun, 2022). Nurses play an important role here as they can involve patients' families in diagnosis disclosure if the patients wish so. Therefore, nurses should be trained to gauge their patients' and families' willingness to talk about EOL matters. This ensures that nurses and oncologists can initiate EOL conversations about advance care planning timely and offer the patients a high-quality EOL experience (Pun, 2022). If needed, considering the family-centred dynamics in Asian EOL contexts, nurses should clarify the roles as well as duties of all the parties in order to foster prompt and accurate decision-making processes.

10) *Breaking down asymmetrical doctor-patient relationships: borrowing the use of open questions from TCM and carrying out in-depth conversations*

   In the context of TCM, holism is fundamental to all philosophies that underlie the practice (Wu et al., 2013). Seeing everything as holistic and integrated allows TCM practitioners to link their patients' existing physical conditions to their former experiences and surrounding environments (Pun & Chor, 2020). The patient-centred discourses embodied in TCM interactions including holism open up the spaces in which patients are invited to offer additional information related to their conditions, giving them the chance to clarify as well as confirm their understanding of the medical information given by their practitioners and feel reassured about their symptoms. Such features of TCM interactions promote more patient-centred care.

   When placed in an EOL context in which doctors play the dominant role, it is helpful for doctors to borrow the questioning skills from TCM practitioners in order to give their patients the space to contribute as much information as they can, and also confirm, clarify or even challenge the information offered by the doctors (Pun & Chor, 2020). Applying various types of questions as TCM practitioners do allows oncologists to elicit their patients' concerns and offer a platform for both parties to create a shared understanding.

In Pun and Wong's (2022) study of TCM practitioners' communication with cancer patients in Hong Kong explored how practitioners build good connections with their patients to reassure them when they are scared and doubtful about their future. TCM practitioners tend to focus on gaining information about their patients' general health conditions in order to develop trust between them (Liu et al., 2013). By laying a solid ground for interactions, TCM consultations with terminally ill cancer patients can turn a lot deeper than those in Western Medicine settings (Pun & Wong, 2022). An interviewed patient noted that such a depth of communication often calmed them:

"I visited TCM practitioners before I visited a conventional medical doctor . . . When the hospital informed me that I needed to receive chemo, I turned to my TCM practitioner for advice. He told me that I must go through the chemo process and I listened. He told me that he understood how hard it is to go through chemo and explained to me that it does not have any side effects . . . When I visit a TCM practitioner, the complete process of consultation is much more detailed. I was asked for a report about my situation and the practitioner took careful notes and gave me suggestions about the whole situation, which made me feel more confident." (Patient M, interview 34)

However, due to the lack of general understanding among patients about TCM practices, such a communication strategy also has its own drawbacks. An interviewed patient said it would be quite challenging to comprehend what is fundamentally going on if one was not familiar with TCM treatments, unlike WM contexts in which most patients tended to have at least a certain level of understanding of the basics of healthcare. That being said, such a problem does not appear to affect patients' understanding of TCM interactions (Pun & Wong, 2022). Some patients explained to the researchers that their practitioner explained TCM concepts to them clearly and in a straightforward manner. Thus, TCM practitioners' communication strategy could still boost their patients' confidence in their healthcare plans and WM doctors could learn from them when facing cancer patients or carrying EOL care in general:

> *"During the whole treatment process, the TCM practitioner's explanations were quite clear. Although we were not informed about the functions of the traditional herbal medicines, we did not need to know this information. All we know is that TCM helped me after my operations. (Patient G, interview 35)*
>
> *Whenever I visit a TCM practitioner, the consultation is always much more personal and well-communicated because I always see the same doctor, unlike in conventional medical consultations, where I may need to see different doctors who tend to quickly finish our conversations. It gives me confidence to know that my TCM practitioner is tracking my health care and helping to control my illness. However, if you do not know anything about TCM, what a TCM practitioner says may not make much sense. In that case, a conventional medical doctor would offer a clearer explanation." (Patient N, interview 33)*

To conclude, the integration of diverse cultural philosophies and religious beliefs plays a fundamental role in shaping end-of-life (EOL) communication in Asian contexts. While Chinese patients and their families generally view death as a natural part of life, their specific attitudes towards dying are deeply influenced by Confucian, Taoist and Buddhist traditions. These influences contribute to the notion of a 'good death', which emphasises dignity, family involvement and the avoidance of unnecessary suffering. As discussed in this chapter, such cultural perspectives present unique challenges for oncologists and palliative care providers, who must navigate complex familial dynamics, societal taboos and patient reluctance to discuss death. The reluctance of both clinicians and families to disclose terminal diagnoses, rooted in traditional beliefs that discussing death may bring bad luck, further complicates EOL communication. Given these challenges, culturally sensitive and family-centred approaches are essential for improving EOL discussions and ensuring that patients' values and preferences are respected.

By drawing on traditional Chinese medicine (TCM) communication styles and integrating culturally tailored frameworks, clinicians can foster more effective and compassionate EOL conversations. Strategies such as indirect communication, shared decision-making within families and structured communication models tailored for Chinese contexts can help bridge the gap between patient needs and medical practices. Ultimately, the goal is to enhance the quality of life for terminally ill patients while easing the emotional burden on their families and caregivers.

Building on these discussions of EOL communication in oncology and palliative care, the next chapter shifts focus to communication challenges in neurology. In particular, Chapter 5 explores how neurologists navigate difficult conversations, such as breaking bad news, discussing prognoses and managing expectations for patients with neurodegenerative diseases. Given the increasing recognition of patient-centred care in neurology, the chapter will also examine strategies for improving patient comprehension, shared decision-making and the role of technology in enhancing neurologist-patient communication in multicultural and multilingual contexts.

5

Neurology

The significance of communication in neurology: Asian contexts

According to the webinar notes of 'Managing Your Healthcare: Communication between the Primary Care Doctor and Neurologist' (Parkinson's Community Help, 2022), it is challenging to coordinate care with neurologists in existing healthcare systems. Therefore, it is important for patients to be informed of how their primary care doctors and neurologists communicate and for different medical departments to make good use of newly developed communication systems including patient portals (Parkinson's Community Help, 2022). In order to ensure that their patients are ready to deal with future illnesses, it is essential for neurologists to be familiar with many communication styles in palliative care such as advance care, learning patients' last wishes and prioritising their physical as well as psycho-emotional needs, delivering prognoses and discussing goals of treatments (Zehm et al., 2020; Boersma et al., 2014; Creutzfeldt et al., 2016). Unfortunately, it remains an issue that neurologists rarely receive enough formal training in palliative care communication (Schuh et al., 2009; Creutzfeldt et al., 2009; Dallara, 2014; Harris et al., 2016; Carver et al., 1999; Mehta et al., 2018).

We interviewed a neurologist based in Hong Kong about patients' communication needs in neurology. In addition to the previously mentioned communication styles, the doctor emphasised the role of family and the importance of addressing doctor-centred communication issues through two-way interactions in Asian contexts:

> *"all the principles of empathy, compassion, et cetera, I think if you can remember about stepping into their shoes and trying to sort of understand what the patient is undergoing, and what the caregiver is undergoing, and what they would like to know, I think this would be the main principle.*

So for effective communication I think a lot of communication is a two way process, so I think we have to engage the patient and the family, and I think effective communication is when they fully understand what are you trying to tell them and you also get a sense that they understand, of course we will need to ask them if they have any questions and so on.

An ineffective communication is when it is very one-sided, the doctor for example dominates the conversation, it also goes the other way around, the patient or the family dominates the conversation, but there is no, I mean, in terms of the interaction, or in terms of the understanding, in terms of mutual understanding of what is going on, I think it may not be very effective."

Recognising the need for neurologists particularly those who work in Asia to receive formal communication training, this chapter offers insights from neurologists in Hong Kong to first identify existing challenges, including the delivery of diagnoses and prognoses, helping patients and their families understand their conditions and carrying out shared-decision-making processes. It then discusses various Asian cultural expectations in neurologist-patient communication in Hong Kong in terms of health literacy, power dynamics, EOL care and the use of tele-neurology. Eventually, communication strategies and technological tools for neurologists based in Asia are suggested to help them explain medical conditions to patients, manage patient expectations, improve patients' health literacy, break bad news to them, involve them in the decision-making process to maximise their quality of care and fulfil their specific physical as well as emotional needs.

Communication challenges and key factors: Neurologist-patient interactions

Delivering diagnoses and prognoses: Being empathetic vs delivering effective treatment in time

While neurologists understand that being able to communicate medical information is a core skill and their responsibility, they face conflicting thoughts on a daily basis: Should they inform their patients of their opinions, which risks receiving angry reactions from them and the breakdown of trusting doctor-patient relationships, or shy away from conversations about psychiatry in order to avoid conflicts and slowly raise more acceptable to gradually convince the patients to receive effective treatment? (Kanaan et al., 2009; Wessely, 1999). It is particularly difficult for neurologists to deliver diagnoses of conversion disorder.

Kanaan et al.'s (2009) study found that neurologists thought it was important for them to adapt their communication style to their patients' receptivity to psychological thinking during this type of difficult conversation. While they acknowledged the significance of being empathetic, the prioritisation of therapeutics over honest medical advice could potentially affect the accuracy of the diagnoses, which minimises the role of psychology and neglects possible symptoms of feigning (Kanaan et al., 2009). According to a surgeon's perspective in our interview, disclosing diagnoses and prognoses to patients without impairments can be even more challenging:

> *"The easiest cases to explain are those where the patient is already experiencing some deficits. Because of these symptoms, the patient can more easily understand that the tumour is affecting their bodily functions and that treatment or surgery is necessary."*

Many other neurologists find it most difficult to break bad news as it can take away patients' hope (Anestis et al., 2021). Not only that they have to deal with their patients' emotional reactions but also their families. All these make it hard for neurologists to involve their patients as well as their family members in the process of decision-making (Anestis et al., 2021). As shown in Anestis et al.'s study (2021), it is quite concerning that over one-third of the participants had never been trained to develop skills to address their patients' emotional needs. While a lot of patients in the EOL want to receive honest information from their clinicians, they still wish to see hope (Clayton et al., 2007). Therefore, it is crucial for neurologists to strike a balance between maintaining hope and giving accurate diagnoses. To do so, neurologists need to be trained to recognise varying optimistic yet realistic forms of hope and convey so to their respective patients and their families based on the patients' communication preferences and focus on what they can do for their patients (Clayton et al., 2007). Another neologist in our interview expressed a similar view when discussing the delivery of bad news to patients in Hong Kong, adding that it is important for neurologists to let patients know that their neurologists and other parties, including nurses and psychologists, are there to be supportive:

> *"rather than concealing any information, I think its important to let them know as much as possible, but I think it's also important at the same setting to provide support and because once they receive the bad news, obviously of course they'll be in shock, but it's very important to let them know that as medical professionals we are doing our very best to help and we are a team of professionals, not only us medics, but in terms of nurses, allied health workers, psychologists, social*

workers, we're there to help as much as possible, and if they need we're always there, available."

On the other hand, from our interview data, perhaps surgeons adhered more to the Chinese authorial communication style for doctors when explaining medical concepts and convincing their patients and their families to follow his advice. However, one surgeon in our interview data still stressed the importance of being empathetic and psychologically preparing them for the disclosure of diagnoses:

"So at times, we have to take care of patient with acute condition, which means that acute deterioration if we not operate at this moment then patient will die. Or have a severe deficit. For this kind of situation I will say that, actually most of them, most of the relatives, members, they will just follow what doctors say, because we would explain to them it is life-threatening condition. If not operate then he or she would die very soon."

"[. . .] to break bad news, because I have to understand for breaking bad news and you may also know that there is a Kübler-Ross model, that is 5 stages of griefs, then every patient or every relative they will have, at a different stage, some at anger, some at bargaining, depression also. So usually I would, first set up a very comfortable, quiet environment and I will also have a tissue ready and then would start to talk about, with all the family members involved and then slowly and also bit by bit. Then I would prepare by studying all the clinical information and then would also try to get some hints from the clinical information system about the background, and then I will talk to them with empathy."

Managing patients' and their families' expectations before making shared decisions

While trained neurologists acknowledge that prognoses are the key moments to implementing patient-centred care and forming effective shared decisions, they are still reluctant to make these difficult conversations (Ahalt et al., 2012). Schenker et al.'s (2011) study found that clinicians involved in EOL care tended to lack the skill to formulate and discuss medical predictions. There are existing guidelines for prognosis disclosure for general healthcare workers and those who specialise in palliative care. However, the area of neurology appears to lack any relevant established guidelines (Glare & Sinclair, 2008; Clayton et al., 2007). In our interview data, doctors shed some light on this unexplored area by sharing their thoughts on managing expectations prior to decision-making processes in the context of Hong Kong. Before making any informed decisions, one doctor in our interview data admitted that he found it particularly important to manage patients' families' expectations when the patients are unconscious as their families would be making decisions on behalf of the patients:

> *"especially from my specialty, I need to communicate well with my patients, because usually my patients usually would be, most of the time have acute deterioration. So I need to have more explanation to have with the family members, rather than the patients, because usually the patient would not be conscious to communicate with. So with those communication with the relatives, they can know more about the diseases and also have a reasonable expectation on the patient outcome, which is very important for subsequent management."*

One neurologist in our interview data further explains that it is a key skill for neurologists to be able to lower expectations and be realistic:

> *"If a patient deteriorates all of a sudden, you did not preemptively tell them about the possibilities. Preemptively, I think this is again another skill which is important."*

Therefore, one of the key factors in neurologist-patient communication is to estimate and communicate 'what to expect', which is unfortunately inadequate in the discipline (Holloway et al., 2013). Due to the lack of communication training, neurologists tend to avoid stating accurate treatment expectations as they do not want to destroy hope (Christakis, 1999; Lamont & Christakis, 2001; Christakis & Iwashyna, 1998). However, contrary to most neurologists' belief, studies have shown that clinicians' dishonesty with expectations will emotionally hurt the patients more (Holloway et al., 2013). Therefore, neurologists need to face the challenge of delivering prognoses and learn to carry out honest and empathetic discussions while managing expectations.

Formulating treatment plans based on shared decisions with patients and their families

As noted, one of the major issues of neurologist-patient communication in Asian contexts is the lack of patient involvement during decision-making processes and diagnostic consultations. The area of neurology has also been identified as a discipline that demonstrates a rather low patient involvement when setting treatment goals and symptom assessment (Christ et al., 2023). One surgeon in our interview expressed the significance of effective multi-party communication to decision-making processes:

"For communication I think it involves, usually involves two parties, or multi-parties and I think having effective communication first, the one who expresses the message, the ideas, must be able to express him or herself first."

Another doctor in our interview further found it crucial for neurologists to understand patients and their caregivers' body language in order to ensure that they understood the provided medical information:

"So I think certainly, of course we have to look into for example, the body language, whether they are nodding or frowning or in sort of confusion. I think this is important, body language is very important when you talk to the patient or family caregivers, whether they understand what is going on."

According to Stern et al.'s (2018) study, most neurologists failed to discuss a range of possible treatment options with their patients, leading to them making decisions without involving the patients. Such a problem continues to exist in medical contexts, which is not ideal as shared decision-making processes allow all parties to fully make use of the best available evidence (Elwyn et al., 2010; Stiggelbout et al., 2012). Neurologists can then also understand their patients' treatment goals and personal preferences, thus fulfilling their needs when choosing the best options (Stern et al., 2018). While some believe that patients would rather let their doctors make decisions on their behalf, Chewning et al.'s (2012) systematic review demonstrated that the majority of patients desired to actively participate when making treatment decisions.

Asian cultural expectations in neurologist-patient communication

Varying levels of health literacy: Tailored discussions

When explaining medical conditions, neurologists find it more difficult to help their patients and their families comprehend the multitude of treatment decisions that come up when these parties are less familiar with neuro illnesses (Zehm et al., 2020). The varying levels of health literacy are often decided by the patients' social backgrounds in Hong Kong as shared by one doctor in our interview data:

"Because everyone has different social background, education backgrounds, some different language skills."

"And then for the receival part of the listener, he or she must be able to comprehend what you say, and because of different social, education background, then we have to tailor made what we talk to them, so to achieve a goal."

As a result, it is important for neurologists to tailor the conversations using appropriate language in accordance with their patients' level of health literacy, including using layman's language instead of medical jargon, which will be discussed in a later section on communication strategies.

EOL care: Making Chinese patients accept reality

Extending on the previous discussions about the challenge of being honest with their patients when carrying out difficult conversations, doctors explained that it was best for the patients if neurologists could convey accurate judgements directly to them and set realistic EOL care goals:

"But for doctors, we have to see all these different kinds of cases many times. So we have to recognise this discrepancy in understanding and have to tell them actually, we tell them our perspective, he or she is likely to be staying like this, almost permanently."

However, he continued that neurologist could show care for their patients by communicating step-by-step through different means such as making phone calls and having a few meetings. He believed that this would gradually help the patients come to terms with reality and make the best decisions for themselves, which in turn enhanced the quality of their EOL care by managing their expectations in terms of recovery:

"So, just need to have many different phone conversations, meetings, and slowly prime them, and then eventually hopefully they will accept, then will accept the condition and accept our suggestion in management.

So at times we have to discuss with some end of care planning, and because like stroke patient, he or she become comatose after the injury, then usually they will kept intubated, which means it would have all kinds of artificial life support: ventilator, some inotropes, some tubings. But then we know that the brain will likely be severely affected, he or she cannot be awaken again. So we have to discuss with them what would be the plan if his or her life cannot be maintained in those critical situations.

Then we have to, there is an option to do CPR (Cardiopulmonary Resuscitation), but then for our perspective, actually all those support may not have very, a lot of benefits."

Doctors found it particularly challenging to accept the likeliness of being unable to recover fully and making EOL plans due to cultural beliefs. By trying to convince the patients and their families to choose treatment options that facilitate EOL care planning, neurologists risked being deemed to have given up on their patients:

> *"But for Chinese patients, because of the culture, it is difficult for them to accept extubation, because whenever you extubate, remove the ventilator, all those support, which means that we are abandoning him or her, not treating her and just ignore them, and to just let them die.*
>
> *For me, at this stage, I still feel not easy, difficult, to talk to them to remove the ventilator, because whenever you tell them we are not sure if extubation, after extubation he or she may deteriorated rapidly or status quo, just keep the same situation. So whenever there is risk of deterioration, they will not accept the extubate."*

If the patients did not raise their advance directives actively, neurologists would often avoid discussing relevant topics like organ donations for fear of angering them and their families as they often refused to accept the likely deaths:

> *"But we will not talk to them for organ donation, even if he or she having brain death, unless the patient has advanced directive, and also unless the family member is very very well accepted the clinical situation, which is not common.*
>
> *Usually they will still in a stage of, sometimes maybe anger, sometimes bargaining stage, so they will not be able to accept what you talk about, so usually I would just let the other organ donation nurses to talk to the family, without any conflict of interest.*
>
> *Because when I talk to them, the family members when they still at the bargaining stage, they will think that we are not treating them, we will just let the patient go and get all their organs.*
>
> *So usually we will, most of the time, ninety-nine percent of the time, we will not talk to the patient about organ donation."*

Based on these observations, it appears that a lot of neurologists in Chinese contexts are aware of the cultural elements that lead to their patients and their families' refusal to make EOL care plans and advance directives, including the taboo subject of death. However, they are not trained to face such situations and would simply avoid confrontations by leaving these to be dealt with by nurses. Due to their lack of skill in making EOL care plans with their patients, neurologists are unable to fulfil their patients' dying wishes and give the best care they can have in the EOL stage. Therefore, it calls for the need to develop appropriate communication training tailored to these cultural contexts.

Communication strategies in Asian contexts

Facilitating patients' understanding of medical issues

Avoiding the use of medical jargon: Speaking in layman's language and analogies

As stated, neurologists in Hong Kong find improving patient understanding crucial to the communication between the two parties. One of the suggested methods is to avoid using medical jargon to help them learn their conditions and avoid misunderstanding in multicultural contexts:

> *"Sometimes may not be your mistake, just they cannot understand or comprehend what you talk about.*
>
> *Because at times there will be some complaints, merely because they cannot understand what you talk about."*

Instead of using overtly complicated medical terms when explaining conditions to patients, especially those from less advantaged social backgrounds, doctors in our interview recommended the use of layman terms tailored to the patients' respective backgrounds:

> *"For me, when I approach the relative, I will, my personal preference is look at where they live, I'm not saying that I am discriminate or do some prejudice on preoccupation, but it is a bit of information that I will know, what is the rough education level of the patient, relative's background, so I can better tailor my communication to a more layman level.*
>
> *[. . .] when it is a problem, usually it occurs both at the grass root patient/relative and also appends to those affluent families or well-educated.*
>
> *For the grass root or less educated relative/family members and he or she cannot comprehend, cannot understand what you talk about, no matter how you say, it is not uncommon, because for my cluster, there's a lot, majority of people usually not well educated or maybe those educated will seek a private medical attention.*
>
> *And I have to use a lot of layman terms and very layman metaphor to let them understand, but after all, usually how well you prepare, how well you communicate to them, they still cannot understand so sometimes I would just let us do our jobs and we would keep communication so would update them."*

Doctors agreed with the use of layman's terms when communicating with patients and their families:

> "I think if you sort of give them too much information, too much medical jargon, then they cannot translate it easily."

He further recommended using analogies to explain to patients and their families bit by bit to enhance their comprehension of medical conditions:

> *"Using analogies is also quite useful, I also always use examples, day in and day out examples when I sort of talk or convey complex problems to our patients and caregivers, so they can relate to what is going on.*
>
> *So sometimes I use analogies, it is like your blender in your kitchen, if your blender, you sort of press onto different speeds, 0 1 3 2 4 at different speeds, then it will not blend nicely and it will form curves, so on and so on, and if you imagine this is the heart, if it was not beating regularly, then clots can form in the heart, but then obviously if these block any blood vessels, then obviously there can be detrimental consequences."*

Practising multilingual communication and translating between languages in a multicultural neurological setting

A key aspect of neurologist-patient communication in Hong Kong is the multicultural nature of the contexts. It means that neurologists in Hong Kong need to be ready to accommodate the patients' native languages to ensure precise delivery of medical information:

> *"So Hong Kong is a multicultural, multi-ethnicity background. So we have to come across many patients speaking different languages, so of course to talk with them, we have to master the languages, but then but of course it is not that easy.*
>
> *Yes I think certainly in Hong Kong, a very, in terms of culturally, a very diverse and obviously Cantonese would be the main modality of communication but we are seeing more and more patients speaking Mandarin, right obviously English."*

Doctors found it important for neurologists in Hong Kong to be able to speak Cantonese, English and Mandarin:

> *"it would be helpful if one would be familiar with Mandarin as well. Certainly we all will be very good with Cantonese and English, but for Mandarin we are using this more and more often."*

When neurologists fail to speak the patients' first languages, doctors suggested getting help from translators to translate complex medical concepts into simple chunks of explanations:

> *"There are also cases, not frequently, but every now and then, patients for example, may not know any English, nor Cantonese, nor Mandarin. Patients from other ethnic minorities, Indian, Bangladesh, Nepalese and so on, sometimes you might need to get a translator in.*
>
> *I think the skill there is to take things very very slowly. You cannot go nonstop, and keep talking, you really have to break down the messages in small chunks, into very very simple messages, and then ask the translator to tell them or to back translate."*

However, there are instances in which the hospitals cannot offer translation services to every patient in need. One doctor shared his experience in using a translation app to communicate with a Vietnamese patient:

> *"And in Hong Kong, in the public hospital setting, we can have interpreter to talk to them, but I have quite personal experience in talking to a Vietnamese patient few months before.*
>
> *Because nowadays I think that technology really helps, in that I use, I ask for interpreter help, at the same time, because I think interpreter cannot be here frequently to explain to the patient. But then I open a social media account, a Vietnamese app. At the same time I use some translation app, then I just communicating with my phone, because I can translate my phone and then communicating with the social media.*
>
> *Although it is not ideal, I think in this age of social media, it is quite helpful for the translation."*

Therefore, it appears that it is worth it for the medical sector to invest more in technology that facilitates translation and thus multilingual exchanges between neurologists and patients, which in turn also alleviates the issue of the lack of manpower in terms of interpreters, especially in a multicultural city like Hong Kong.

Increasing health literacy and encouraging access to support

To offer the best quality of care for patients, neurologists need to be able to explain all the treatment options. One of the barriers, as stated, is the low level of health literacy among the public. Therefore, neurologists perhaps can help their patients and their families access medical resources by telling them what to expect and what alternative support they could seek when diseases cannot be treated:

> *"And then we tell them what to expect from the patient, and also I have to tell them what to expect when they need to take care of them, because the patient may be dependent, which they need a lot of personal care, assistance.*
>
> *other than the caring part, for the disease part, then I ought to tell them what are the alternatives and options they can do. And sometimes, our ability is limited, we cannot treat all the diseases. Then I have to introduce to them what others, psychological support, religious support, then he or she may be able to approach."*

By offering such information upfront before the patients' conditions deteriorated, neurologists could manage patient expectations and avoid any backlashes from their families, as stated by one doctor in our interview data:

> *"If you can preemptively give the patient or caregivers all the information upfront, then if a certain complication comes out, they'll not be taken by surprise, because we have already mentioned it as a possibility."*

The doctor also found that neurologists would mentally prepare the caregivers for unfortunate situations by enhancing their level of health literacy:

> *"So I think lowering the patients and relatives' expectations is very important, otherwise they may not expect certain things to come through. But then if you already told them okay every step what is going on, I think that also helps psychologically.*
>
> *if something did complicate the illness, I think the chances of, I mean, complaints, or unhappy family members would be lower."*

The neurologists therefore have to offer ALS caregivers in particular accurate resources to facilitate their understanding and sort out the information the caregivers found on the internet, and then help them interpret the obtained resources (Newham et al., 2006). In turn, this should allow the neurologists to gain the patients' and caregivers' trust and improve patient compliance (Chiò et al., 2008).

Training neurologists to break bad news: Empathetic patient-centred care

As previously discussed, neurologists should learn to promote a sense of hope and be prepared to break bad news. One doctor in our interview data stressed the significance of striving for a balance between making the patients feel optimistic while managing realistic expectations:

> *"Then I would prepare by studying all the clinical information and then would also try to get some hints from the clinical information system about the background, and then I will talk to them with empathy.*
>
> *I have to know all those information in order to make them feel comfort, but at the same time we cannot talk very optimistically, have to be cautiously optimistic."*

The dimension of empathy is key to neurologist-patient communication according to our interviewees. Pepper et al.'s (2022) study also states that a sense of empathy and positivity during diagnoses is the key to successful treatments. This would essentially build mutual trust between neurologists and their patients, leading to patients' willingness to communicate their preferences and needs. Therefore, effective communication can facilitate the implementation of patient-centred care as neurologists form individualised treatment plans tailored to the patients' needs by addressing their most prominent presenting core and non-core conditions (Pepper et al., 2022).

Training courses: Systematic neurologist-patient communication

In general Chinese contexts, scholars like Yao et al. (2023) have observed the need to improve neurologists' communication skills by advocating the implementation of systematic and professional neurologist-patient communication training sessions. Yao et al. (2023) found neurologists' communication skills often inadequate, which could not be solved by the accumulation of their clinical practice. It is essential for them to be aware of how they can review the next steps with the patients, proactively invite the patients to raise matters that they would like to discuss and clearly explain the rationales for the suggested diagnostic procedures (Yao et al., 2023).

The rising use of tele-neurology in the post-Covid era: Where does future neurologist-patient communication lie?

As shown by the earlier experience of using a translation app and social media with a Vietnamese patient, there is a trend of utilising technology to facilitate neurologist-patient communication. One doctor in our interview data explained that the use of tele-neurology has particularly spiked since the pandemic, aligning with Klein and Busis' (2020) findings:

"So during COVID, the main problem is that the patient–relative cannot visit the patient as before.

The only way to communicate would be either by phone conversation, or now we can have some video calls to communicate with them.

And for my specialty, as mentioned before, the patient will be very dependent, then relative may not be able to understand or expect right at the date of admission. Then I have to keep on using phone to communicate and if possible, arrange the video calls, so let them to see the patient. Because some patient, the relative expect after the operation, some will expect the patient will get conscious again, can communicate."

Assisting their patients to communicate with their family members when they could not meet face-to-face allowed neurologists to demonstrate care for them:

"I think I mentioned its important to again step into the shoes of our patients and caregivers. COVID-19 has impacted because caregivers cannot visit the hospital, nor can they visit the elderly homes, and then so on.

I think sometimes just by acknowledging or telling the patients and caregivers, telling them you know it's a very very difficult time, and these sort of words I think, does help with easing or providing some comfort.

in terms of using other means of communication, be it video conferencing, facilitating this as much as possible through allied health workers or social workers, or even sort of, even if these may not be available.

even taking the chance when we're speaking to the family members, I mean on the phone. And sometimes just handing the telephone to the patient, so at least they have a brief moment of communication, and moment with loved ones, I think that already means a lot to the family members and the patient."

These changes have since then influenced society in the longer term. Some neurologists find that tele-neurology can help build a stronger sense of community, improve population health and the quality of care for patients as well as lower costs for multiple parties (Klein & Busis, 2020). However, tele-neurology has only been widely used in recent years as a specific audio-visual means of communication. It requires several aspects of support, including authentic engagement and rapport, appropriate placement of healthcare providers and patients, suitable room layouts, adequate non-verbal communication skills, effective documentation, as well as time management (National Consortium of Telehealth Resource Centers). Therefore, it takes time for hospitals to train neurologists to be familiarised with the technology and use it effectively.

To conclude, this chapter has explored the communication challenges neurologists face in Asian and multicultural medical contexts, including dominant family-centred values, the authoritative role of doctors, a lack of empathy, delayed diagnoses and prognoses and limited patient involvement in decision-making. By incorporating original interview transcripts with neurologists in Hong Kong, this chapter has provided insights into the underlying cultural expectations in Asian neurological settings, including the varying levels of patients' health literacy influenced by socio-economic backgrounds, the taboo surrounding death and the complexities of planning end-of-life (EOL) care. Based on these first-hand findings, communication strategies tailored to Asian and multilingual contexts have been proposed, such as leveraging language and translation tools, providing patients and caregivers with access to both physical and mental support and implementing structured training programmes on breaking bad news and improving neurologist-patient communication.

Moreover, the rise of tele-neurology in the post-Covid era presents new challenges and opportunities for enhancing neurologist-patient communication. While future research may contribute to the development of more sophisticated communication technologies, hospitals and medical educators must proactively design training programmes that ensure the effective and culturally sensitive use of these tools. As we transition to the next chapter, we shift our focus from neurology to surgery, where communication plays a crucial role in ensuring patient safety and shared decision-making. In surgical contexts, communication breakdowns can lead to critical errors, complicating both pre-operative consultations and intra-operative teamwork. The following chapter will examine how surgeons in Hong Kong navigate these challenges and implement strategies to enhance communication in high-stakes medical environments.

6

Surgery

Introduction: Surgeons' communication challenges and the significance of effective communication

While there have been great advancements in the area of surgery, complications still occur frequently because of preventable human errors. Miscommunication tends to be a key cause of these errors (Etherington et al., 2019). When failing to coordinate and communicate effectively, surgical clinicians are likely to cause higher mortality rates and more post-operative pain with lowered functioning levels for their patients (Mills et al., 2008). Unlike other clinical contexts, the errors made in operating rooms are relatively more catastrophic, which might lead to scandals for surgeons and their affiliated institutions (Makary et al., 2006). Miscommunication in an operating room can result in wrong-site/wrong-procedure surgeries, retained surgical sponges, unmonitored blood transfusions, mismatching organs for transplants and neglecting allergies. With effective communicative systems, these errors could be prevented. According to a study reported by the Joint Commission on Accreditation of Healthcare Organisations (JCAHO) (1998), ineffective communication was one of the most common root causes of sentinel occurrences and wrong-site surgeries. Therefore, surgeons and hospitals need to build a culture of effective communication to ensure patient (Makary et al., 2006). From global observations to the case of Hong Kong, this chapter zooms in to reveal communication challenges faced by worldwide and particularly Asia-based surgeons and includes original advice offered by local doctors during their interviews with the authors' team on tackling Chinese cultural expectations during pre- and post-surgical communication and complications in the surgical setting of Hong Kong.

Inefficient team communication

To achieve high-reliability teamwork in operating rooms and surgical wards, clinicians have to be able to monitor each other's performance, implement effective team leadership and team orientation, learn to back each other up when cooperating, adapt to the fast-paced environment, build mutual trust and establish shared mental models (Etherington et al., 2019). Only by doing so, the team would be functioning well and capable of delivering quality treatment and ensuring patient safety (Tørring et al., 2019). As a doctor in our interview spoke to the author's team, coordinated care is crucial to guarantee the level of complexity of the surgical procedures performed:

> *"I think it is very crucial and indispensable, because we are work as a team, so without communication, then definitely we cannot work."*

A lot of studies demonstrate that surgical teams that communicate well exchange more medical information among members when compared to those that do not (Westli et al., 2010; Mesmer-Magnus & DeChurch, 2009). However, while this correlation is rather well-established, Cumin et al. (2016) carried out a simulation study and found that the participants failed to share relevant medical information 48 per cent of the time, especially when it came to scrub nurses, anaesthesia technicians and surgical trainees. As a result, communication breakdowns happen a lot in operating rooms. Hu et al.'s (2012) study even showed that these errors happen every seven to eight minutes, particularly during exchanges between professions. Ninety per cent of these incidents would lead to negative consequences to the surgery, including delay, procedural error, resource waste, team tension, near misses or even adverse events (Hu et al., 2012; Kripalani et al., 2007).

Language barriers: Obtaining consent from patients

Another key communication challenge surgeons face is interactions with patients (Chan et al., 2019). They usually encounter barriers during pre-operative consultations and obtaining informed consent from their patients. This is due to the nature of the urgency and emergency in the area of surgery. There are many instances in which surgeons find it impossible to discuss the patients' situations with them in detail (Chan et al., 2019). In a case reported by Chan et al. (2019), a surgeon could only gain informed consent from hospital administrators because they failed to be in touch with the intubated patient's next-of-kin in Australia about them needing a procedure to be done.

Time constraints and noisy environments in busy surgical settings

Considering the nature of the environment in surgical wards and operating rooms, the complexity, dynamics, time constraints and life-threatening instances also negatively impact the effectiveness of communication (Gillespie et al., 2013). It is necessary for surgeons to master verbal forms of interactions as they are significant for them to understand each other's meaning, particularly in ad hoc teams in which team members do not know one another well (Osborne-Smith & Hodgen, 2017). This is because clinicians in intra-operative teams are usually required to multi-task and wear masks that conceal most of their faces, making it difficult to communicate through non-verbal cues like facial expressions (Osborne-Smith & Hodgen, 2017). The emotional stress would potentially facilitate communication breakdowns (Osborne-Smith & Hodgen, 2017). Therefore, considering the constraints of non-verbal communication in operating rooms and surgical wards, surgeons need to recognise the important role of effective verbal communication.

Moreover, environmental factors such as noise in operating rooms and busy surgical wards can lead to case-irrelevant dialogue at the expense of case-relevant discussions (O'Daniel & Rosenstein, 2008; Osborne-Smith & Hodgen, 2017). Studies have shown that such irrelevant communication like social talks would distract and even disrupt tasks that concern surgical procedures and anaesthesia tasks, which could potentially result in negative patient outcomes (Healey et al., 2006; Sevdalis et al., 2007; Schiff et al., 2016). Other than non-essential small talk, frequent interruptions like phone calls, pages, personnel entering and exiting the room as well as bedside teaching can also compromise effective communication (Gillespie et al., 2013; Healey et al., 2006).

What does effective communication entail in the context of surgery in Hong Kong?

Ensuring patients' understanding of surgical processes and goals: Empathetic verbal communication and health literacy

A doctor in our interview shared that it is important for surgeons to understand that communication is a two-way process. Messages must be delivered and received clearly to achieve mutual understanding, especially when interacting with patients who have different social and educational backgrounds:

> *"For communication I think it involves, usually involves two parties, or multi-parties and I think having an effective communication first, the one who express the message, the ideas, must be able to express him or herself first.*

And then for the receival part of the listener, he or she must be able to comprehend what you say, and because of different social, education background, then we have to tailor made what we talk to them, so to achieve a goal."

A doctor in our interview noted similarly and added that surgeons should respect their patients as equals. He found it helpful to step in the patients' shoes before communicating and acquire the skills of listening to the patients despite the time constraints:

"So, I think, to myself, communication has to be at least two ways, the recipient/our opponent and ourself. We need to have some degree of equality actually, not that we are doctors and we are more superior. We actually have to respect our patient and try to stand in their shoes and to think of how they perceive the information that we are going to convey to them. I think there are a few obstacles that will hinder effective communications. For instance, listening. Actually, it is a very simple word but a lot of people miss and also overlook the importance of listening. Not just use our ears to listen to patients but actually we need to also put down everything that we have on our mind. Our own agenda, sometimes in a business clinic, they will think that the time is running out in the out-patient clinic and we have some other chores to do, like the emergency operations and so on. We actually have to put that down to really listen to what the patient is going through."

Also, a doctor in our interview explained the importance of avoiding the use of medical jargons. Otherwise, patients would struggle to understand:

"And another obstacle is the verbal communication, I think, which is how we convey our message. Especially, as doctors, we know a lot of jargons, medical jargons, which are very complicated and a lot of concepts that are actually inconsiderable by patients. Actually, we have to make it really simple and easy to understand."

A doctor in our interview further elaborated that surgeons to be aware of the patients' level of health literacy as it would affect how they perceive the illnesses. It would take time for patients to digest the bad news, so it is important for surgeons to be empathetic while efficiently deliver medical knowledge in a quick and concise manner in order to facilitate the decision-making process regarding surgeries:

"Another problem is perception actually because how we perceive the disease is different from how the patient perceive the disease. Usually, the patient first knowing that they have cancer, they will be really shocked and they will go through a few faces in a while, anger, depression and so on. While our own agenda is to convey the message to them as fast as possible and to let them know that you need

surgery or surgery is not useful to you, we have to use the shortest amount of time to tell them about that. Actually, that's quite disturbing because the patient will perceive the disease as the end of the world while we are actually treating it as a day-in day-out normal encounters so how we perceive the disease is actually very important. And also, we need to actually think of how the patient think about their disease and try to look at the disease through their eyes and address their concerns."

Pre- and post-surgical care: Reassuring patients

For surgeons in particular, it is crucial for them to reassure their patients during pre-surgical discussions and post-surgical care. A doctor in our interview noted how he paid special attention to post-operative patients as they would wake up being uneasy. Therefore, he found it necessary to fully explain how the surgeries went and manage their expectations about recovery, discharge timelines and when they would be able to resume daily routines:

"Especially, I pay more attention in time on our postoperative patients. For example, I will try to explain to them what happened in the operation whether it is smooth or not, and our expectation on their recovery time, and when they can be discharged, and when they can resume their feeding and drinking and so on."

Before surgeries, a doctor in our interview stressed the significance of obtaining consent from patients and ensuring that they understood the risks and medical implications. This is crucial for patients to manage their expectations and digest the relevant and possibly overwhelming information:

"Another group of patients that we always spend some time on is our preoperative patient that were admitted for the preparation for the operation. So, usually we will already have the consent signed in the out-patient clinic. It's our routine to talk to them again about the risk and also the whole procedure so that they have a better understanding because there is usually a lot information to take in during the busy out-patient clinics. So, usually they need some time to digest and formulate their questions and their concerns. So, usually we will spend more time and talk to them about the expectation management whether or not they have the stoma, for example."

Timely DNAR decisions and sensitive delivery of bad news

One of the surgeons' key tasks is to make Do Not Attempt Resuscitation (DNAR) decisions in a timely manner with the patients and their families. A doctor in our interview noted that it would not be easy as patients and their families found it difficult to accept, so surgeons must facilitate efficient decision-making processes by offering their medical analyses:

> *"But for surgeons, the DNAR actually is another very important topic that we have to cover it because usually we have a patient coming in through emergencies and sometimes, we need to DNAR the patient in a very short period of time. For example, we have a patient with rupture aortic aneurysm. He was very old so he does not fit for any surgery and rupture aortic aneurysm is fatal in a matter of hours, if not minutes. So, we have to tell the patient's relatives as well as the patient that they have this kind of disease that we cannot help and they will die in a very short period of time. So, it's actually very difficult for them to accept, especially for patient with this kind of disease, they usually were well and enjoying their lives and suddenly it's like a bomb and it goes off and they are in the hospital and in the next hours or minutes they will probably be dead or they may lose their lives. That's the very difficult situation that we need some time to encounter."*

A doctor in our interview acknowledged the difficulty of carrying out sensitive conversations about end-of-life (EOL) care, particularly when patients and their families are unprepared for such news. In some cases, as he described, patients arriving at the hospital were unaware that they were already suffering from terminal illnesses. Consequently, receiving a sudden diagnosis of advanced cancer was often shocking and emotionally overwhelming for both the patient and their relatives. This emotional distress made it even more challenging for doctors to discuss do-not-attempt-resuscitation (DNAR) decisions and the shift towards palliative care. The doctor explained:

> *"Another problem that we also encounter is the patient with advanced cancer that came in but was not diagnosed before. For example, a patient comes in with abdominal pain and we did a CT scan and showed that there is a disseminated colon cancer with a lot of metalepsis to lung, to liver, and so on. And also, it's obstructed so the patient actually had an emergency situation, but there's actually little that we can do to help him. So, we also need to see all the relatives as well as the patient to let them know what's going on, and we need to tell them that if the patient finally deteriorates, we will not resuscitate. So, the art of telling them not to resuscitate when the patient experiences cardiac arrest is quite difficult sometimes. But what I usually do is I tell the patient's relatives that they have – or the patient has – an incurable disease and will die in a short period of time. So, we are trying to make them feel comfortable and will try to give them symptomatic treatments."*

As the doctor emphasised, framing the discussion in a compassionate and supportive manner is crucial. Instead of using medical jargon or alarming terminology, such as 'resuscitate', which could be misinterpreted as giving up on the patient, doctors focus on explaining the goal of maximising comfort and minimising suffering. The challenge lies in ensuring that families understand the medical reality without feeling abandoned by healthcare providers. The doctor elaborated on his approach to DNAR discussions:

> *"For DNAR, what I usually do is to tell the relatives of the patient that they have a disease that may take their lives in a short period of time. And we are trying to give them symptomatic treatment and try to make them comfortable. The very important thing is not to use the term 'resuscitate' because it's very irritating to the patient, or even the relatives. If you say, 'When the patient has cardiac arrest, we will not resuscitate,' then it seems like we are not doing our job or that they are not doing their job, their own responsibility."*

This statement highlights the cultural and emotional complexities surrounding EOL discussions in medical settings, particularly in contexts where families play a central role in decision-making. Many relatives struggle with the idea of DNAR, fearing that it equates to withholding care. To navigate this, the doctor carefully rephrases his explanations, reassuring families that while certain aggressive interventions – such as chest compressions and intubation – will not be performed, other forms of medical support will continue. He further explained:

> *"Our aim is not to cause any more pain to the patient and let them go peacefully. So, what I usually tell them is that we will not do these two procedures – chest compression and intubation – when there is cardiac arrest. But all other treatments, for example, antibiotics and infusion, we will still provide to the patient, as well as oxygen."*

By framing DNAR as a decision to prioritise patient comfort rather than as the withdrawal of care, doctors can help families accept the inevitable outcome with greater understanding and less distress. This approach underscores the importance of empathetic communication, particularly when discussing terminal illnesses and EOL care.

As medical professionals continue to refine their communication strategies, training in delivering bad news and discussing palliative care remains essential. In the next section, we explore how these communication challenges extend to surgical settings, where high-pressure environments and time constraints often complicate doctor-patient interactions.

The case of Hong Kong: Chinese cultural expectations

Reaching consensus and managing expectations with patients and their families

As previous chapters have highlighted, the role of families is key to medical communication in Asian Contexts. When it comes to surgeries, it is particularly crucial for surgeons to reach a consensus with not just the patients but also their relatives. Sometimes, there are chances that adverse effects might occur during surgeries. It is also not guaranteed that surgeries will be successful. Therefore, it is important for patients and their families to understand the risks involved and surgeons should manage their expectations regarding operative risks and effectiveness of the suggested surgical plans very carefully with patience and time, just as a doctor in our interview data suggested:

> *"Another problem that may arise is actually the difference between our own expectation and the patient. For example, we have a case of Ischemia. It means poor blood supply to the bio due to blockage of the blood vessel. So, the bio becomes dead. In that case, we had a patient with this problem but at the same time she had background diseases of metastatic bone disease and also an aneurysm in her forensic aorta so actually combines with the patient's age, which was 86. So, she was old and her operative risk was very high but her disease may need surgical intervention if they wanted to be cured and go home. So, we had to actually discuss with the patient's relatives and the patient a lot, using a lot of time and a lot of patience to tell them about not going through the operation or whether or not we should go through with it because there is a high possibility that the patient may die on the table due to not just the disease itself because the patient had a very high operative risk. So, it's that time when the patient's relatives convey to us that they didn't expect the patient to go so suddenly without any treatment, especially when the patient was actually well and about a few days ago before admission to the hospital, she could walk around and actually do her own chores and her daily activities. They didn't really expect the patient to come in with something that could not be cured and then the patient would probably die in the hospital. It's all about communication with relatives and sometimes not just communication skills but we also need time for the patient's relatives and the patience to accept that some diseases cannot be cured or some diseases will take their lives eventually."*

Caring for patients' emotional needs during diagnoses and the role of families as comforters

It is not uncommon that patients fail to emotionally process the diagnoses of their terminal illnesses. It is not easy for Asian patients to feel comfortable communicating their feelings to medical professionals that they barely know. According to a doctor in our interview data, they would feel more reassured after seeking social support from their relatives. Therefore, he suggested that surgeons should advise patients to take as much time as they could before making a sound decision or even going home and discuss with their families before the next consultation:

"I could think of there was one time that we had a patient with colorectal cancer. We were in the out-patient clinic and tried to tell them about the disease. They really couldn't take it. Actually, they got really emotional and angry at the same time. They thought the doctor missed the diagnosis in the early disease stage. Also, when we are trying to discuss operation to them, they feel like information overloaded. They are actually unable to process anything at that time. How we dealt with that is actually we terminated our meeting and we told our patient that it's okay and I know you need a few minutes or even a few days to process what's going on and we totally understand and we will see you again, maybe next week with your carers, your relatives so they will have their social support as well as other people that can listen to what's going on. They can supplement that to the patient."

Communication strategies for surgeons in Asian contexts

Being empathetic to and comforting patients by explaining medical knowledge through multimedia tools

As a doctor in our interview previously stressed, it is very important for surgeons to be empathetic in order to show their support to their patients. It is difficult for patients to mentally process that they are suffering from terminal illnesses. Therefore, surgeons should comfort them and offer them options to deal with the situation:

"For listening, I have actually mentioned quite a lot that we need to address the patients and not just address the patients' problems and concerns, we also need to be empathetic. We need to show our empathy to the patient that actually having a cancer is bad, but it's not the end of the world and there are actually a lot of things that we can do to eliminate that or even cure it."

A doctor in our interview also recommended using not just simple language but also visual tools like diagraphs, pamphlets and videos to enhance patients' understanding of their medical issues and what to do when feeling discomfort:

"For verbal communication, usually we will need to use simple words that I have mentioned and drawing diagraphs and also sometimes we make use of pamphlets

that we prepare or videos. We actually have quite a number of videos, teaching the patient about what to expect when they have a stoma. For example, how they should take care of the stoma and how it would look like, which position it would be at."

Creating a safe space for patients to digest information in the busy clinical settings of Hong Kong

As stated, surgical wards are often very crowded, especially in the settings of Hong Kong. This means that surgeons have limited time dealing with each patient and have difficulties concentrating due to human noises. Therefore, a doctor in our interview said surgeons should arrange for case nurses to communicate with the patients about their emotions and medical issues, and even set up a hotline to support patients under stress and answer their queries. This way, the surgeons can compensate by offering patients emotional support as consultations are usually cut short:

"Also, for time factor, actually, during the out-patient clinic, we have a lot of distractions and we are running out of time. There are noises around and there are people in the next consultation room. Next-door people can be very distracting to a patient. Sometimes, we will have a separate consultation by the case nurse. We have a dedicated colorectal nurse to actually counsel on the patient, address their problems. Patients have a hotline to call when they are in stress and when they have further questions. That actually helps us, doctors, a lot because we don't have a lot of time sometimes to explain to patients of what to expect. Usually, we just cover the risk and indication and about the operation but not a lot the patients' feeling. It actually helps if we can spend more time with the patients but in reality, it's difficult."

Loop communication in busy surgical wards

In the field of healthcare communication, close-looped communication is regarded as one of the most effective communication strategies in operating rooms (Etherington et al., 2019). Surgeons worldwide tend to adopt this structured communication protocol and standardised terminology and procedures: the communicator who initiates would give a message (the call-out), and then the receiver repeats it back to confirm the accuracy of the message, and the initiator eventually re-confirms the message is correct to close the loop (Härgestam et al., 2013). One of the doctors in our interview suggested strategies is loop communication as well, particularly during peak hours when things are hectic:

"So, one of the peaks for communication with other colleagues is doing emergencies when everything is so messy. It happens so fast and usually we make use of loop communication. Loop communication means that when we give an order, for example we give certain drug, we will yell it out loud and also address it to a specific person. For example, nurse A, please give this patient drug A, fifty milligram through iry access. And then the nurse A will feedback to me as saying the same information that we will ensure that we are giving the patient the right drug, and right amount and the right type and the right administration way. So, this is one of the important things that we have in loop communication and also very important during surgery. And during surgery, it is very important to keep in contact with our enlicises because for example, when the patient had torrential bleeding, we will need to inform our enlicises earlier for them to prepare, for example, prepare some blood transfusion as well as some resuscitative drugs. And when the patient has some problems, for example, with intubation during the procedure, during the operation, the enlicises will also inform us that the patient's acceleration is coming down. So, we need to terminate our operation at this moment or we have to temporary stop the operation to figure out what happens to the patient before going through or the patient now is crashing, so we need the shortest period of time to do damage control surgery to complete the surgery in the shortest period of time and as soon as possible."

A doctor in our interview has illustrated example which proves that loop communication ensures the efficiency, accuracy and precision of communication, which is essential to the implementation of efficient information transfer in a dynamic setting like the operation room (Härgestam et al., 2013). Moreover, the strategy of loop communication is straightforward and does not cost hospitals extra, making it a very ideal strategic solution to miscommunication (Schuenemeyer et al., 2017). That being said, the use of the strategy in the operating room has not been extensively researched, even though it has been proven to be useful in improving patient safety in non-operating settings like surgical wards. Therefore, researchers should investigate how loop communication can be developed into intervention designs to be employed in real-life operating settings (Etherington et al., 2019).

Gradual bad news delivery: Drawing on the surgeons' experience, the use of empathetic language and role-playing practice sessions

Like medicals in other disciplines, bad news delivery is challenging to surgeons. A doctor in our interview suggested a gradual delivery to ease the patients' shock. For instance, he would explain the background of the patients' symptoms and essential medical knowledge before discussing the diagnoses. After that, he would stress what the surgeons could do for them according to his experience, instead of making the patients fixate on the bad news itself:

> *"For delivering a bad news, it is actually of an art. It takes experience to actually deliver the message to the patient or the relatives. So, usually what I do was to set the scene first. So, I sit them down comfortably and I try to introduce the whole background and the condition of the patient first before delivering that bad news. So, usually I will say, for example, Mr. Chan. He was last time admitted for some abdominal pain and we did something, some investigation for him, for example gonospy and we found a tumour. So actually, I just went through with the flow and then I start to slowly give out the information about the bad things that the patient had a tumour. I will tell them that we found a tumour. We are not sure whether it is a tumour or not. So, we took some biopsy and we are still waiting for the result or we have the result now. It's actually cancer. So, I will usually paraphrase with what we will usually do for our other patients, not just this patient so that we can actually make the patient to feel like they are not the only one. We actually have a lot of experience on this and they can rely on us. So, I will tell them that usually for a patient with colon cancer, we will do certain imaging to see the disease progress and whether we can do surgery to reset it or not. So, usually the patient will be more accustomed to what we are trying to tell them because we are releasing it slowly and naturally but not telling the patient that I got bad news for you."*

To help surgical students develop the skill of showing empathy to patients and their relatives and consequently build rapport with them, a doctor in our interview recommended that they practise through role-playing sessions as these would allow them to step into others' shoes and learn to cope with various challenging situations:

> *"a very important aspect of communication is not just the knowledge. You actually have to be empathetic to the patient. Also, be professional so the patient or the relatives can trust you. So, how to be empathetic? I usually teach my students or the young doctors that you pretend that your patient is your relatives or even yourself and then try to think in their shoes and try to think what they are going through before actually starting a conversation with them or trying to bring your bad news. So, actually the mental preparation on that can help you with the delivery of the bad news and also to establish a better rapport with your patient. And how do I teach them sometimes is, one of the ways is to do role plays. So, role-playing is very important. Usually, we have two students doing it. One pretends to be the patient*

and the other one, the doctor. So, what they are trying to do is that one tries to convey the bad news to the patient, and the patient tries to be a difficult patient, so tries to act out, tries to be emotional and sees how they cope with that."

Moreover, a doctor in our interview added that instructional videos would be an effective way to show students good and bad examples of bad news delivery:

"Another way is to show them videos of how it should be done, how we actually tell our patients when they have terminal disease or so on, and also bad examples that may potentially badly influence the relationship between the patients and the doctors"

Facilitating communication between patients and their loved ones through technology

In the post-Covid era, surgeons have begun to continue using technological tools like online video calls to facilitate communication between patients and their families as the patients could still gain emotional support from their close ones who lived remotely:

"So, COVID-19 actually causes some problems. One of the problems is that we cannot see the relatives of the patient that easily because of the risk of infection and the patient's relatives actually could not sometimes visit their loved ones when they are hospitalised. We try to deal with that by not just calling their relatives by phone but also make use of Zoom or other apps that we can get our hands on to let the relatives see the patient's face and actually communicate with the patient and that we can also, at the same time, convey the patient's current condition and plan through the Zoom meeting."

To conclude, families play a crucial role in communication between surgeons and patients in East Asia, particularly given the emotional distress patients experience and their occasional inability to make decisions due to unconsciousness. Miscommunication in these high-stakes settings can delay essential DNAR and surgical decisions, putting patient welfare at risk and, in extreme cases, leading to fatal outcomes on the operating table. This case study of Hong Kong highlights the importance of effectively communicating medical information and providing reassurance to patients before and after surgeries in busy surgical settings. Such communication is vital for reaching shared decisions among patients, their families and medical professionals.

While strategies such as loop communication, technological tools, the creation of safe communication spaces and role-playing exercises have been adopted by surgeons in Hong Kong to support patients emotionally, further research is needed to evaluate the effectiveness of these strategies in real-life surgical environments across East Asia. Moreover, as medical professionals continue to refine their communication approaches, training programmes should integrate these findings to enhance doctor-patient and interprofessional communication in surgical settings.

As we transition to the next chapter, the focus shifts from surgical communication to the role of nurses, who often serve as intermediaries between doctors and patients. The following chapter examines the cultural nuances of nursing communication in Asia, the challenges of working in multilingual settings and the strategies nurses employ to facilitate patient-centred care, including active listening, non-verbal communication and culturally competent approaches to end-of-life discussions.

7

Nursing communication

Researching Asian-specific features and adapting to cultural norms in nursing communication

Effective nursing communication plays a crucial role in patient-centred healthcare. When efficient communication occurs between nurses and patients, patients tend to be more content with the care and comply more with the medical regime. Moreover, good nursing communication can also foster therapeutic rapport, have positive impacts on patient care and avoid negative medical incidents (Afriyie, 2020; Kourkouta & Papathanasiou, 2014;). It is important to recognise that nursing communication in non-Western contexts also requires nurses to be proficient in intercultural communication, especially in the culturally diverse contexts of Asia. By emphasising the values of cultural distinctions, nurses can enhance their patients' treatment and master communication in a wide range of clinical settings (Claramita & Susilo, 2014; Zayts & Kang, 2010).

Recognizing the intercultural aspect of nursing communication outside the Western context, this chapter focuses on the necessity to incorporate Asia-specific features in the said research area. Firstly, it is crucial to realise the importance of cultural sensitivity and linguistic diversity. Douglas (2011) suggested nurses to follow twelve standards of practice for culturally competent nursing care, including (1) social justice; (2) critical reflection on their values, beliefs and cultural heritage as well as their impacts on culturally congruent healthcare; (3) gaining sufficient knowledge of cultures, including family systems, community practices and other traditions; (4) implementing culturally competent practices by applying their intercultural knowledge; (5) acquiring the cultural competence in healthcare organisations and systems, meaning that their institutions should offer the structure and resources essential for nurses to evaluate and fulfil their diverse patients' cultural and language needs; (6) being familiar with the concept of patient advocacy and empowerment, and consequently advocating for the inclusiveness of their patients' cultural values in existing healthcare systems; (7) ensuring a multicultural workforce; (8) delivering and receiving communication training that promotes culturally competent nursing care; (9) using cross-cultural verbal and non-verbal communication skills to understand patients' beliefs, perceptions and healthcare needs; (10) performing cross-cultural leadership to guide their teams to offer competent care for their diverse patients; (11) participating in the process of healthcare policy development; (12) reading evidence-based research and then implementing effective communication strategies when communicating with patients from different cultural backgrounds as well as investigating how disparities in healthcare outcomes can be solved (Douglas, 2011). We can observe from Douglas's (2011) research that nurses and researchers should aim to understand their patients from different angles, including language, religion, customs, cultural traditions, their respective socio-economic backgrounds and levels of health literacy in order to design holistic care (Betancourt, 2006; Nápoles-Springer et al., 2005; Ayonrinde, 2003; Epner & Baile, 2012). Only by achieving cultural competence, nurses can build trusting relationships with their patients and thus improve healthcare outcomes as patients will be approached in ways that are congruent with their cultural values and norms (Douglas, 2011).

This chapter also suggests ways for nurses to adapt communication practices to regional values and norms. For instance, insights from our interview data with local clinicians highlight the importance of language adaptation, including the use of key phrases and greetings in patients' mother tongue, avoiding medical jargon and incorporating interpreters or translators when necessary. Additionally, clinicians emphasised the role of non-verbal communication, such as recognising patients' non-verbal expressions and adjusting interactions to align with regional norms, including respecting personal space, time orientation and culturally hierarchical structures that shape patients' communication styles and other norms (Chan, 2011; Kim & Oh, 2016).

Characteristics and challenges of nursing communication in Asia and Hong Kong

Literature review on historical and current practices: Core cultural values and the lack of cultural-specific communication models

Jin et al. (2002) presented a few well-rounded case studies of cultural and clinical issues encountered by Asian patients in their care, including language barriers, socio-economic gaps and varying health belief systems and practices. They noted that nurses should not make cultural assumptions about patients' heritage and should instead plan treatments collaboratively to accommodate patients' needs (Jin et al., 2002). Moreover, Jin et al. (2002) also urged nurses to acknowledge cultural differences, use translators when needed, understand their use of alternative treatments like Traditional Chinese Medicine (TCM) and research their patients' cultural backgrounds. For example, as illustrated in the introductory chapters of this book, nurses should be familiarised with the degree of collectivism or individualism that their patients are accustomed to in terms of the level of family involvement and personal autonomy in healthcare decision-making; the level of power distance, the degree of hierarchy, respect and deference that patients and nurses show to each other and other healthcare professionals; patients' orientation towards high-context or low-context communication such as how much patients and nurses rely on explicit verbal messages or implicit non-verbal cues to convey and interpret meaning; the influence of traditional health beliefs and practices, i.e. TCM concepts.

While there are existing communication frameworks and models for nurses worldwide, there is an absence of culturally appropriate models that differ from the Western ones. As a result, there is a great challenge as the lack of Asian-specific models limits the applicability of current strategies to local clinical practices and patient expectations (Pun et al., 2018). Even though former literature has drawn connections between nurses' perceptions of the CARE (connect, ask, respond and empathise) model and ISBAR (introduction, situation, background, assessment, recommendation and readback) protocol and the degree of medical information they gain during communication, there is still a lack of research that extensively elaborate on how to implement these strategies to maximise the quality of nursing care, especially during handovers (Andersson et al., 2014). Moreover, while Pun's 'Nurses' perception of the ISBAR handover protocol and its relationship to the quality of handover: A case study of bilingual nurses' (2023) has strived to fill in the research gap of bilingual verbal communication during nursing handovers and the use of ISBAR protocol, there is a limited focus on non-verbal and contextual cues as well as the integration of traditional communication values and norms within established models (i.e. TCM and spiritual care) that influence the effectiveness of nurse-patient communication in a lot of Asian clinical settings (Liu et al., 2005; Lam et al., 2020; Tiew & Creedy, 2010). Therefore, the following sessions cite the interviewees to understand Asian-specific communication challenges in nursing communication through the case study of Hong Kong.

Language barriers in multilingual settings

In bilingual Asian settings like Hong Kong, healthcare professionals tend to interact using both their mother language and English to carry out medical information exchanges, which could result in a complicated communication process of 'code-switching' or 'translanguaging' that are hard to monitor and susceptible to errors (Pun, 2021; Pezzolesi et al., 2010). These language barriers to healthcare would even pose more threats to patient safety within trilingual emergency rooms as constant code-switching and translanguaging can easily lead to miscommunication (Al Shamsi et al., 2020; Pun et al., 2015b; Pun, 2022). A clinical professor at one of the Universitiesin Hong Kong we interviewed has highlighted the language gap between healthcare professionals and their patients in Hong Kong as they receive education in English, but Hong Kong is a bilingual society, making it important for them to learn medical terminology in Cantonese or Chinese as well:

> *"Sometimes you also have to equip yourself better by looking up different terminologies in different languages, we are taught in medical school mainly in English but we are largely a bilingual society in Hong Kong so it's also important to understand or learn some of these medical terminologies in Cantonese or Chinese as well."*

She further stressed the significance of practising commonly used languages in Hong Kong:

> *"I think again if you are particularly fluent in one language and not in others it can be said that you have to practice, practice and practice. You have to practice in speaking in the languages you are not most comfortable with so for me it might be speaking in Mandarin which sometimes now have to do with the changing composition of the population so for you it might be another language, but really try to practice and not be scared of using languages you might not be most familiar with."*

By being familiarised with different languages, nurses can minimise the difficult and complex switches between medical language in English and everyday language in Cantonese or sometimes Mandarin, which consequently lowers the chance of communication failure with patients in a multilingual environment.

Cultural nuances that influence the nature of nurse-patient interactions

Cultural stigmatisation: Gender dynamics and prejudices towards patients

In Asia, there is an asymmetrical relationship not only between doctors and patients but also between nurses and patients (Ishikawa & Yamazaki, 2005). As per Wang (2010), Chinese patients tend to be used to playing a submissive role when interacting with healthcare professionals. As a result, conversations become centred around healthcare professionals and lead to patients' dissatisfaction since there is often a long waiting time for rather brief consultations (Yin et al., 2012). Such a cultural phenomenon has caused negative impacts on other aspects of patient experiences too, including gender dynamics. In Hong Kong, female patients reported being awkward when having to speak to their male medical staff about symptoms related to overactive bladders, making them feel like they have no option at all when selecting medical treatments (Siu, 2015). As Hsiao et al. (2006) discussed, the traditional role of men in Chinese cultural contexts had made male healthcare workers less empathetic (Hsiao et al., 2006) as patriarchal ideologies did not encourage men to be expressive, thus leading to ineffective communication (Attree, 2001). In addition to that, patients suffering from psychiatric disorder are also less likely to seek help due to their experience of stigma when speaking to nurses and doctors about their medical issues in Hong Kong (Mak et al., 2015).

Time constraints and high-stress environments

In the specific cultural context of Hong Kong, time is considered a critical variable when implementing quality nursing communication (Chan et al., 2012). An oncologist we interviewed has explained that everyone, including patients and their families, is busy in Hong Kong, which makes communication challenging as stakeholders are easily distracted due to the crowded settings:

> *"In my opinion, lack of time is certainly the most important thing. Interestingly, not only doctors are busy, but also family members. Another problem is the setting. As you know, Hong Kong is crowded with people everywhere, and hospitals are no exception. It is difficult to achieve good communication when the place is either too crowded or with a lot of distraction and noise."*

The cultural taboo of EOL discussions

A local oncologist we interviewed has highlighted another key cultural nuance in Chinese hospital settings, namely the taboo of speaking about death-related issues. She stated that patients' families played a major role in her past communication with patients about EOL care and that they tended to hide timely news from the patients, which negatively impacted patient-nurse communication:

"Be sensitive when communicating death-related issues and give hint first/ and invite consent before you proceed [. . .]. Collusion is common in Chinese culture – we usually explore reason why they want to hide the news from the patients, make sure the family understand hiding essential information from the patient can make patients more stressed, and reassure them you will do this gently. Family takes important role in decision-making. [. . .] be sure to involve close family members Be sensitive to family dynamics, identify carer stress, identify and invite key-person for decision making."

Two doctors we interviewed have both thought and noted the importance of revealing all essential with honesty but also addressed the challenge of not appearing to be blunt in order to let the patients and their families digest the news:

"Rather than concealing any information, I think it's important to let them know as much as possible, but I think it's also important at the same setting to provide support and because once they receive the bad news, obviously of course they'll be in shock, but it's very important to let them know that as medical professionals we are doing our very best to help and we are a team of professionals, not only us medics, but in terms of nurses, allied health workers, psychologists, social workers, we're there to help as much as possible, and if they need we're always there, available."

Wang and Chan's (2015) systematic review of EOL care research in Hong Kong noted a similar concern as it demonstrated that local patients who did not have a clear sense of their prognosis were more likely to feel anxious and experience challenges when interacting with their relatives.

A doctor we interviewed has further found that the family-centred values in Chinese contexts made it hard for him and the nursing team to convince the families to do what would be best for the patients, especially when it meant ending their lives:

"for Chinese patients, because of the culture, it is difficult for them to accept extubation, because whenever you extubate, remove the ventilator, all those support, which means that we are abandoning him or her, not treating her and just ignore them, and to just let them die. For me, at this stage, I still feel not easy, difficult, to talk to them to remove the extubation, because whenever you tell them we are not sure if extubation, after extubation he or she may deteriorated rapidly or status quo, just keep the same situation. So whenever there is risk of deterioration, they will not accept the extubate. And then, there is also an issue about organ donation, because I will say many of the patient suitable for organ donation will be from my specialty or neurology related to the brain, because usually for the brain, acutely injured brain patients, then usually other organs are well functioned."

According to Wang and Chan (2015), such a problem leads to 95 per cent of informal caregivers in Hong Kong encountering difficulty when caring for their family members in the EOL stage as they have inadequate medical knowledge and skills to make the best decisions during palliative care. This would potentially lead to emotional distress because they feel that they have not fulfilled filial responsibilities (Chan et al., 2015). Therefore, it is important for nurses to be equipped with the cultural knowledge relevant to EOL care and for hospitals to offer supportive programmes for both healthcare professionals and family caregivers (Wang & Chan, 2015).

Tackling nursing communication challenges

Active listening and tailored emotional support: Filling in the gap of nurse-patient communication

A nursing professor at one of the universities in Hong Kong shared a key concept that she learnt from nursing school that would lead to mutual understanding and thus effective communication, which is active listening:

> *"I would say effective communication is difficult. When we are talking about communication, we normally tell people how to actually speak, how to talk to the patients, what are the information that you need, what will be the content of the communication. However, the most important thing, or the most challenging thing is active listening. Listening actually play a very much important role in communication. So not just only talking, but also listening. I still remember when I was an undergraduate in here, at the school of nursing of XXX University , teachers actually taught us about active listening. I would say at that time, just the term 'active listening', I don't think, at that time, I was able to do that because when we are talking about active, we really listen to patients, we really understand something behind the patients, something that they didn't tell us. But we understand. So, active listening is, if we are very, very skilful in active listening, probably the communication is much more effective."*

Due to the doctor-centred culture in Chinese contexts, an obstetrician-gynaecologist we interviewed has stressed the crucial role of nurses as 'good people' as they would often be the key healthcare workers to offer emotional support to the patients after active listening:

> *"Patients do not want to express too much emotion in front of us, so nurses can sometimes be good person to express some of their negative emotions."*

In challenging periods like the pandemic, nurses' communication with families is important as they can offer reassurance while listening to the relatives' concerns:

> *"For our patients who are unconscious our nurses give a daily update to the relatives at the minimum. We have to constantly remind ourselves of the difficulty of the relatives in not being able to follow a disease progress it's really hard to come to decisions with regards to treatment. So we really have to interview them take proactively on a daily basis in order for them to have the best picture with regards to updated condition on their patients."*

A nursing professor we interviewed has further highlighted the significant role of nurses as doctors would frequently rely on information that emerged from nurse-patient communication due to time constraints:

> *"in terms of nursing, especially as a nurse, I think communication is very important because we have to handle patients daily. And we also need to communicate with different disciplin*
>
> *es in the hospitals like doctors. We always need to communicate with them because we are the ones that, for twenty-four hours, we are beside of patients. But doctors normally will have very minimal time spending with them. So, we have to tell them about the patients' progress and also patients' needs, and also, we need to take care of the carers. There are a lot of things that we need to communicate."*

Moreover, each patient has their own concerns, meaning that nurses have to tailor the conversations and try to understand them before taking any medical actions for patient safety, as per the interviewed doctor said:

> *"Normally in nursing, they need to do, and give very simple and clear instruction. But sometimes, for nurses, as I've said, nurses are always in the ward for twenty-four hours, and we are there because patients have different problems. Every single patient is unique. Even though they have the same diagnoses, they have different kinds of problems or difficulties. We are the persons that are trying to help the patients to solve the problems. Whenever the patients tell us the problem, we are trying to listen, and then trying to understand, and trying to clarify what they are actually telling us. So, this is the meaning I have to make sure I receive the correct message before I act anything. I think this is also important."*

Understanding non-verbal cues and body language to tackle language barriers

A local doctor we interviewed has stated that there are some symptoms that do not allow the patients to articulate themselves clearly, including physical disabilities like dementia and other factors like depression and language barriers, so she would teach the team to use tools like cue cards and search for non-verbal cues:

> *"Some of the patients may not be able to speak clearly. Say for example, people after stroke, or like the dementia patient, sometimes they cannot really express very clearly. So, not only just listen to patients but also try to look at their nonverbal cues. For example, not only just physical disabilities but sometimes for patients with depression. They don't want to talk. But if they are admitted with some of the problems, we understand them just because of some nonverbal cues, facial expressions for pain, or sometimes their preferences. So, looking at the patient's face is also very important. Or sometimes, people in ethnic minority group, they can talk but somehow, they cannot express very well in terms of the language. We don't understand their language as well. So, it is talking about body language, it is talking about trying to listen to what they are talking about. Even though we don't understand, sometimes we also use cue cards, the cards having some pictures and words, and trying to communicate. Of course, there are interpreters in hospital authority, we can use that kind of services. But for immediate response or immediate communication, normally these kinds of things can help."*

Delivering bad news in person

After going through the hard times of the pandemic, a doctor we interviewed has acknowledged the challenge of being unable to break bad news face-to-face as nurses could not observe the patients and their relatives' emotions and reactions. Therefore, a doctor from our interview recommended in-person conversations instead of phone calls:

> *"Telling the patient or the carer the bad news is really challenging. Especially during covid 19 pandemic, no visitation currently. If the patients have condition deterioration, it is quite difficult to talk to the patients or talk to the patients' carers. I would say this really need some of the very skilful communication. Normally, when we break the bad news, we would like to break the bad news face-to-face because you understand the person that receive your message and you're trying to help, you're trying to intervene different kinds of emotions at the same time. However, during covid 19 pandemic, no visitation. If there is any deterioration of the patients, we don't really just call the patients through the phone. Using phone to break bad news is very challenging. Normally at this moment, we would just try to give very simple communication, and try to ask the patients' relatives to come to the hospital first. Then we do everything afterwards. So, breaking the bad news face-to-face is much better."*

Culturally competent communication training programmes

A number of programmes have been launched to promote cross-cultural competence in multicultural healthcare settings. They offer a variety of practical tools for nurses to learn the influence of cultural differences on nursing behaviours and enhance the development of new forms of cross-cultural collaborations between nurses, patients, caregivers and doctors. It is important for researchers and hospitals in Asia to introduce the aspects of multiculturalism during medical education and nursing training programmes, which is especially crucial in global institutions in which intercultural skills are not an advantage but part of the normal way of nursing in multilingual settings like Hong Kong (Xu & Davidhizar, 2005).

Implications and future research trends in nursing communication: The applications of technology

Emerging trends and issues in nursing communication research are increasingly shaped by advancements in technology. Key areas of development include: (1) the integration of technology, with a growing reliance on telemedicine and digital medical records (Li et al., 2017); (2) the expanding role of artificial intelligence (AI) and machine learning (ML) in medical decision-making, including predictive analytics for patient outcomes, diagnostic support, and personalised treatment plans (Rajkomar et al., 2019); (3) the adoption of health monitoring technologies for secure data management, such as wearable devices for continuous health tracking and telehealth platforms that enable nurses to provide remote patient care (Steinhubl et al., 2015); and (4) the increasing use of simulation-based training in nursing education, including virtual reality applications for surgical procedures and patient safety scenarios (Pun, 2023a).

To conclude, this chapter has explored key communication challenges and the potential impact of implementing new strategies that are unique to nursing communication, not only in wider East Asia but also in the specific context of Hong Kong. Given the doctor-centred communication style prevalent in Chinese cultures, nurses play a crucial role as the primary communicators with patients in daily interactions. In multilingual Asian settings, cultural competence is essential for nurses to effectively engage with patients from diverse linguistic and cultural backgrounds, addressing factors that shape healthcare perceptions.

To navigate the challenges posed by language barriers, time constraints and cultural nuances – such as gender dynamics, cultural stigmatisation of certain diseases, taboos and family-dominated decision-making – nurses must bridge the gap left by limited doctor-patient interactions. This involves practicing active listening, providing tailored emotional support, skilfully delivering bad news and employing non-verbal communication strategies to enhance patient care.

Future research should build on these findings by integrating technological advancements into nursing communication. The development of culturally appropriate AI- driven models could help mitigate intercultural issues, address language barriers and alleviate workforce shortages while fostering more holistic and continuous patient care.

These themes of cultural competence and effective communication are equally critical in geriatric care, where nurses and physicians must navigate additional complexities such as end-of-life discussions, advance care planning and the role of families in medical decision-making. The next chapter will examine how these factors shape communication with elderly patients in geriatric settings, particularly in the context of Hong Kong's aging population.

8

Communication with elderly patients in the area of geriatric care

Introduction: Low literacy in end-of-life (EOL) care

Effective communication plays a crucial role in geriatric care as it is integral for accurate assessment and the formulation of suitable treatment plans for the elderly's complex healthcare needs including multiple chronic symptoms and unique medical goals (Huang et al., 2021). By enforcing good communication, doctors and nurses can build trust with their patients and make sure that the latter's values and preferences are considered when forming treatment plans, which is essential for the improvement of their quality of life as well as their level of satisfaction with their care (Clark, 1995). However, despite the significance of geriatric communication, researchers like Nedjat-Haiem et al. (2013) found that many patients from non-white cultures tend to have less knowledge about End-of-Life (EOL) care choices compared to their English-speaking world due to health literacy, cultural competency and other cultural factors. For example, Chan and Pang's (2007) study in Hong Kong revealed that many nursing home residents tended to be uncomfortable about discussing their preferences for EOL plans in terms of life-sustaining treatment (Pun, 2020). Only the Law Reform Commission of Hong Kong published a consultation paper about substitute decision-making and ADs in 2006 that highlighted doctors' adherence to their patients' AD and EOL preferences. Such an issue is often caused by the East Asian perceptions of viewing death as a taboo subject and patients' families as a key stakeholder in EOL discussions, and the expectation of the patients fulfilling their familial role under Confucian social constructs (Pun, 2020). Therefore, there is an urgent need for geriatric professionals and researchers to understand the cultural differences in EOL communication in order to resolve suboptimal care (LoPresti et al., 2016). Moreover, patients' EOL processes will be greatly improved with less use of the hospital if geriatricians are able to effectively initiate Advance Care Plan (ACP) discussions with patients and their families, which in turn also allows better resource allocation in overloaded medical systems (Norals & Smith, 2015) in contexts like Hong Kong.

It is also important to note that researchers should not generalise Asian contexts as there are cultural differences in geriatrician and patient perceptions as well as EOL communication in various regions like Hong Kong, Japan, Korea and China (Park et al., 2018). Even though these cultures are greatly centralised around Confucianism and the emphasis on the dominant role of the patient's family, geriatricians from these cultures address DNR orders and discuss EOL matters in different manners due to the varying degrees of Westernisation, healthcare systems and economic statuses (Park et al., 2018). Therefore, researchers must bear in mind these factors when evaluating the challenges and forming recommendations for geriatricians to communicate with their patients. The purpose of this chapter is thus to explore the cultural differences in DNR and ACP in Western and Asian contexts through the case studies of Hong Kong and to underscore the importance of such planning for patients' quality of life.

Cultural differences: Varying attitudes towards DNR and ACP in Western and various Asian contexts

The emphasis on patient autonomy in the West

In general, DNR orders are for patients to make clear that they would not like to undergo resuscitation when an unforeseen, irreversible condition occurs and leads to a cardiac arrest (Gelbman & Gelbman, 2008). In the West, patient autonomy is treated as a fundamental premise, especially when it comes to a patient's right to make their own EOL decisions like refraining from any cardiopulmonary resuscitation following a terminally ill patient's cardiac arrest. It is believed that such stress on patient autonomy has successfully promoted AD and thus the quality of EOL care (Eliott & Olver, 2007; Boyd, 2001). For example, several studies pointed out that most patients have CPR preferences and would like to participate in the decision-making process in the United States (Cherniack, 2002; Hamel et al., 2000). It is not uncommon for relatives to misinterpret the wishes of their elderly family members, and even physicians make the same mistake (Liddle et al., 1993; Zweibel & Cassel, 1989; Gramelspacher et al., 1997; Wenger et al., 2000). Therefore, the Western medical discourse focuses a lot on the implementation of optimal utilisation of DNR such as how to apply the ethical principles of patient autonomy and medical professionals' beneficence at the same time (Cherniack, 2002).

Striking a balance in Chinese palliative contexts: Communicating with patients and families in EOL discussions

Chinese and Western cultures perceive palliative care differently and thus have varying expectations (Pun et al., 2023). A lot of Chinese patients trust their physicians and close relatives to make final EOL decisions on their behalf (Bowman & Singer, 2001). According to Pun et al.'s (2023) integrative review, the key factors that affect EOL and palliative decisions in general Asian contexts are family members' wishes and religious beliefs (Wang et al., 2016; Peng et al., 2012; Miljeteig, 2010). The collectivist value rooted in Chinese culture influences patients in the sense that they would rather make collective decisions with their families or in some cases even completely entrust them to make choices (Bowman & Singer, 2001). The core Confucian moral value of filial piety leads to the Chinese elderly patients' belief that their children should naturally understand their personal preferences and thus make decisions on their behalf in the last life stage (Fan et al., 2019; Kwak & Haley; 2005). Unfortunately, such a value also frequently results in collusion, a scenario in which the family tries to hide the diagnosis from the concerned patient in even Western-influenced Asian settings like Hong Kong and Singapore (Pun et al., 2023; Low et al., 2009), believing that such lies would enable the patient to have a 'good death' (Lo et al., 2001). Cases like this hinder the implementation of patient autonomy that is prevalent in the West. Even though many recent reports have demonstrated that medical workers commonly concur that EOL discussions should involve patients and relatives (Almack et al., 2012; Kasbom et al., 2020), studies have shown that Asian patients like those in Taiwan have increasing concern about their level of autonomy when making EOL decisions. For example, the rates of DNR orders and hospice care utilisation had significantly grown between 2008 and 2014 in Taiwan (Shih et al., 2017). Therefore, geriatricians in Asia have to be culturally competent enough to carry out AD discussions with both their terminally ill patients and families effectively in order to promote holistic EOL care (Pun et al., 2023).

The importance of encouraging ACP for patients' quality of life

Ideally, advance care planning consists of continuous discussions and assessments among medical professionals, patients and their relatives. Throughout the process, it is important for clinicians to address their patients' and families' emotional needs, making sure that care goals are prioritised over specific treatment plans (Tulsky, 2005). By encouraging ACP, clinicians can (1) help their patients identify and implement their individual wishes for EOL plans as well as show their respect to the patients, especially when they are unable to make sound decisions when suffering serious illnesses; (2) aid their patients in managing personal matters in a state of peace without burdening their loved ones; (3) reduce stress, anxiety and depression in their patients' relatives; (4) improve patient satisfaction of EOL quality (Lum et al., 2015); (5) ensure that their patients have autonomy in decision-making processes and confirm enduring guardianship (Duffield, 1998; Inman, 2002); (6) minimise medical interventions (Tierney et al., 2001); and (7) decrease their patients' hospitalisation (Kernick et al., 2018). Considering all these benefits of discussing ACP with patients, it is significant for geriatricians and researchers to help promote educational programmes and awareness campaigns (Pearse et al., 2021) as well as be capable of using culturally sensitive materials and approaches to communication with patients (Zager & Yancy, 2011). By achieving the above goals through continuing education on ACP, geriatricians can enhance concordance between patients' EOL wishes and care, including preferred place of death (Pearse et al., 2021).

In multicultural contexts like Hong Kong in particular, individual patients need to be evaluated in relation to their familial and cultural contexts (Zager & Yancy, 2011). Therefore, ACP and AD discussions need to be based on geriatricians' knowledge of the corresponding cultural groups. Clinicians should be able to promote patients' and relatives' understanding of EOL care in diverse cultural settings. More research is needed to ensure that desirable outcomes for patients can be fulfilled in relation to their cultural beliefs and values.

Challenges in geriatric communication in Asian contexts

Language barriers and health literacy

Communication is a significant part of EOL decision-making processes; therefore, patients with language barriers are at high risk for suboptimal decision-making (Barwise et al., 2018). In outpatient settings in particular, these patients risk lower-quality EOL care due to ineffective discussions about goals of care plans and inaccurate understanding of their diagnoses as well as prognoses (Silva et al., 2016; McGrath et al., 2001; Chan & Woodruff, 1999). Numerous recent studies have shown that patients from minority groups tend to have lower rates of AD planning because of inefficient communication due to race, ethnicity, language barrier and culture (Barwise et al., 2018; Kwak &

Haley, 2005). Therefore, it is important for geriatricians to use language that their patients can comprehend and apply any other communication aids when necessary (Mullick et al., 2013). Training programmes should be set up to train physicians to clarify the language employed in these conversations and increase awareness of their patients' preferences which can be contextually fluid based on cultural backgrounds (Deep et al., 2008).

Moreover, limited health literacy has negative impacts on ethnic minorities and the elderly in particular (Periyakoil et al., 2015). This is because they tend to forget most of the medical information conveyed to them and half of the content they remember is inaccurate (Kessels, 2003). They may also be incapable of understanding complex medical concepts including resuscitation preferences (Periyakoil et al., 2015). Therefore, in multicultural environments, geriatricians need to be trained to prevent using medical jargon when interacting with their patients from diverse cultural backgrounds and use tactics such as teaching back to evaluate their patients' level of comprehension of the medical information provided (Schillinger et al., 2003).

Do Chinese patients in Hong Kong really see death as a taboo subject?

As per discussions in previous chapters, many scholars and physicians believe that having conversations about death is a taboo in Chinese societies, especially when dealing with the elderly (Chu et al., 2004). However, Chu et al. (2004) and Wu et al. (2002) discovered that elderly patients in Hong Kong tend to show a relatively lower level of anxiety when facing death and a limited number of them admit that they fear death. Chu et al.'s (2004) study demonstrated that the interviewees were not worried at all about having EOL conversations. Surprisingly, the participants demonstrated good acceptance of discussing deaths and life-sustaining matters. For example, they said they did not feel fear of dying because they already had grown-up offspring, elaborated posthumous plans like funeral arrangements, a good long life and so on (Chu et al., 2004). Contrary to the generalised belief of Chinese patients seeing death as a taboo subject, the studied patients were open about EOL discussions and did not see death as a taboo subject. Interestingly, some even thought it was a relief to speak to their physicians about EOL matters (Chu et al., 2004). Therefore, it is important for geriatricians and researchers to design further studies and extend their services on this area in order to offer holistic care that is culturally appropriate for the elderly population in Hong Kong.

Recommended strategies

Understanding patients and families: Expectations and situations

A geriatric doctor we interviewed has highlighted the significance of not jumping to the conclusion of recommending a DNR no matter how busy the ward is as a lot of communication with the patients' families is needed, so physicians can learn the specific patient's situation and expectations:

> *"I think the first thing is we need to start with the right approach, I think a lot of times, in a busy hospital, when we call up the family for the first time and explain that the patient is very ill and then immediately transition to a discussion about a 'do not resuscitate' order, it jumps over a lot of communication that needs to be happened before we talk about the DNR order. We need to first explore what's their understanding of the patient's illness and what are their expectations, and if their expectations are very far from what really is going on, how ill the patient really is. Then immediately I know that we can't talk about DNR. We need to get on the same page first. And sometimes that takes time for them to build trust and you as the provider, for them to see also that their loved one indeed is very ill."*

Delivering bad news: Choices of words

Since many Chinese people are quite reluctant to talk about their relatives' potential deaths, an oncologist we interviewed has recommended giving cues and gaining consent for EOL discussions to be initiated in order to emotionally prepare patients and their families for the difficult conversations:

> *"Be sensitive when communicating death related issues and give hint first/ and invite consent before you proceed."*

A local surgeon we interviewed has stressed that the key is to carefully choose your wording when speaking about DNR decisions. For example, he would avoid the word 'resuscitate' in order to prevent the patients and their relatives from being upset. Otherwise, some might even think that the medical professionals are refusing to do their job:

> *"For DNR, what I usually do is to tell the relatives of the patient that they have a disease that may take their lives in a short period of time. And we are trying to give the symptomatic treatment and try to make them comfortable. The very important thing is not to use the term 'resuscitate' because it's very irritating to the patient, or even the relatives because if you say when the patient has cardiac arrest*

or permeate arrest, then we will not resuscitate. Then, it seems like we are not doing our job or they are not doing their job, their own responsibility."

Proactive engagement with patients and families: The expression of care

To facilitate the process of making DNR-related decisions in Hong Kong, a clinical professor we interviewed has noted that these could be made easier by early engagement, discussing prognoses, providing comfort, emphasising care and relieving suffering. Most importantly, it is important to show patients and their families that the physicians have tried hard by spending a lot of time to communicate and show care to them:

"So DNR means do not resuscitate. It's a decision we have to make although difficult for a large proportion of our patient who do not respond to conventional or to the best care. Actually I found it not to be as difficult as it seemed to me when I first started. Because I've noticed if you engage in discussion early in their disease progress and you're able to walk the few days however short days spend in the ICU. You walk those days with the relatives then usually they are able to come to terms in terms of the disease prognosis much more easily. If they've seen therapy and the time you have given to their patient relatives. They understand what the disease prognosis is and it's much easier to bring about this discussion of perhaps maybe we have limit the care and if the patient falls apart then not to resuscitate. I think we try to emphasise that it's not a decision of giving up and it's very true, it's really a lot of times the last thing you can do for patients whose disease do not respond to therapy. It's to give them those last few hours of comfort and peace where it's respectful for the patient because they from your medical experience you know that they will probably not respond to resuscitation anyways. So doing that on its own is futile."

Non-verbal cues: Tackling language barriers and understanding hidden thoughts

Given that Asian patients can shy away from discussing their AD and ACP with people outside their families, a nursing professor who we interviewed stressed the cruciality of observing patients' non-verbal cues including facial expressions and even preferences:

"But if they are admitted with some of the problems, we understand them just because of some nonverbal cues, facial expressions for pain, or sometimes their preferences. So, looking at the patient's face is also very important."

By doing so, geriatricians can respond to their patients' emotions, get involved in non-verbal communication and learn more about their patients' present quality of life, desires as well as fears (Piers et al., 2018). Such forms of communication are crucial as the patients' emotions can highly influence their decisions about AD and ACP (de Boer et al., 2012). Afterwards, geriatricians can actively involve the patients' relatives by offering insights into their patients' preferences for care goals and EOL wishes (Dening et al., 2011; van der Steen, 2010; Sampson et al., 2011). In the case of dealing with patients suffering from dementia, geriatricians' observations and interpretations of their patients' behaviours and emotions would be particularly important when aiding them and their families in making EOL decisions (Piers et al., 2018).

Moreover, Hong Kong is home to people of many ethnicities as a multicultural city. Therefore, doctors in our interview note that many languages are spoken and language barriers often hinder effective communication in the hospital, making it important for physicians to understand body language and use tools like cue cards to facilitate mutual understanding:

> *"People in ethnic minority group, they can talk but somehow, they cannot express very well in terms of the language. We don't understand their language as well. So, it is talking about body language, it is talking about trying to listen to what they are talking about. Even though we don't understand, sometimes we also use cue cards, the cards having some pictures and words, and trying to communicate. Of course, there are interpreters in hospital authority, we can use that kind of services."*

The dominant role of family: Considerations of stakeholders

In the area of geriatric care, it is inevitable and significant to involve patients' family members during bad news delivery and decision-making processes. Unfortunately, the impact of family caregivers and companions on the decisions made regarding EOL matters like cancer treatment is usually neglected, despite the fact that families are a substantial influence. As per Clayman et al. (2005), roughly 20 per cent to up to 50 per cent of elderly patients have a designated family caregiver who accompanies them during medical visits. Pun et al. (2023) recommended geriatricians to offer essential information about various possible EOL decisions in order to guide the caregivers in formulating EOL decisions with or for (when the patients are physically incapable of making decisions at all) their dying family member, which is echoed by our interviewed doctors:

"We have a patient with rupture aortic aneurysm. He was very old so he does not fit for any surgery and rupture aortic aneurysm is fatal in a matter of hours, if not minutes. So, we have to tell the patient's relatives as well as the patient that they have this kind of disease that we cannot help and they will die in a very short period of time."

Moreover, the recommendations from doctors in our interview data align with Pun et al.'s (2023) guideline on providing sufficient support and education to the caregivers, alongside addressing their concerns, expectations of care, experiences and fears are they might be unprepared:

"On the second hand, if the relatives are able to come to terms with this decision. They are allowed to sit by the bedside. They get to spend more time in peace and comfort and quiet with the patient. Then we also emphasise that we'll try to keep their passing and pain-free and suffering-free and that really helps. If they are able to understand that medical care or treatment itself is not going to reverse the illness then what we're doing in terms of making the decision not to resuscitate is also care for the patient and that makes the whole decision easier on their part as well."

*

To conclude, this chapter has reaffirmed the importance of Advance Care Planning (ACP) and Advance Directives (AD) in geriatric care, highlighting the cultural differences that shape patients' varying attitudes towards Do Not Attempt Resuscitation (DNAR) across Western and Asian contexts, including Hong Kong, Singapore and Taiwan. While research indicates that Chinese patients are often influenced by collectivist values and cultural taboos, geriatricians in multicultural settings must develop cultural competence to navigate different levels of patient autonomy and tailor their approach based on familial and cultural beliefs.

To address communication challenges in geriatric care – such as language barriers, health literacy disparities, and patient reluctance to engage in end-of-life (EOL) discussions – this chapter has drawn from interviews with clinicians to present effective communication strategies. These include actively understanding patient and family perspectives before discussing DNAR decisions, choosing words carefully when delivering bad news, demonstrating empathy through proactive engagement, utilising non-verbal cues to interpret patient needs and considering familial dynamics in decision-making. Further research is needed to refine culturally appropriate communication strategies and enhance the delivery of geriatric care across diverse Asian contexts.

The discussion of effective communication in geriatric healthcare transitions naturally into the next chapter, which examines multilingual and culturally sensitive communication in veterinary medicine. Just as human healthcare professionals must navigate language and cultural barriers to improve patient care, veterinarians must also develop strong interpersonal and linguistic skills to communicate effectively with pet owners and colleagues in diverse clinical settings.

9

Veterinary perspectives

Multilingual and culturally sensitive communication

The importance for veterinary students to develop communication skills

In veterinary medicine, effective communication plays a crucial role in enhancing clinical outcomes, such as improving client satisfaction during veterinary visits and persuading clients to comply with suggested treatment plans (Artemiou et al., 2014; Englar et al., 2016). Failure to communicate efficiently can lead to health, safety and legal issues for veterinary professionals (Adams & Kurtz, 2017; Kinnison et al., 2015; Kurtz et al., 2017). To promote effective communication, veterinarians need to engage with both pet owners and their animals. Hamood et al. (2014) highlighted that human medical patients place more value on the care and relationships with their doctors than anticipated (Englar et al., 2016; Frankel, 2006). Since then, many medical institutions have worked to address this shift in perspective. It is essential that veterinary schools provide training in communication skills, leading to a growing field of research focused on the interactions between vets and clients, including needs, expectations and results (Bowman et al., 1992; Kurtz & Silverman, 1996; Levinson & Roter, 1993; Maguire, 1990; Makoul, 2001; Smith et al., 1999).

Research has shown that both veterinary professionals and students consider verbal communication and interpersonal skills to be critical in their work (Haldane et al., 2017). However, many practitioners have noticed that recent graduates often lack these essential abilities (Adams & Kurtz, 2017; Bowman et al., 1992; Kurtz et al., 2017; Makoul, 2001). As Dickinson et al. (2011) observed, many participants in their study felt they needed further postgraduate training to improve their skills in clinical communication (Kogan et al., 2004). These insights underscore the importance of veterinary medical schools equipping students with communication skills, preparing them for the varied challenges they will face in real veterinary practice (Kinnison et al., 2015). Integrating these components into the veterinary curriculum will help ensure that new professionals are better prepared for clinical situations.

A lot of veterinarians find communication skills essential, with some considering them an aspect of clinical competency since effective communication can greatly improve the precision and effectiveness of their work (Englar et al., 2016; Hamood et al., 2014; Kurtz et al., 2017; McDermott et al., 2015). These insights suggest that interpersonal abilities and communication techniques play a major role in building rapport with clients and fostering positive veterinarian-client relationships (Adams & Kurtz, 2017; Kurtz et al., 2017; Rösch et al., 2014). As a result, communication training is viewed as a critical part of veterinary education and is required by the American Veterinary Medical Association (AVMA) and other accrediting organisations in many regions and countries (Gaida et al., 2018).

Although veterinary communication has been extensively examined in Western contexts, there is a growing need to investigate how culturally influenced communication skills are developed by veterinary students in non-English-speaking regions (Pun, 2020a; 2020b; 2020c; 2020d). To create communication models that are culturally relevant for Hong Kong's veterinary students, this chapter discusses Pun's (2021a; 2021b; 2021c; 2021d 2023a; 2023b; 2023c; 2023d) projects that focused on assessing the communication needs of these Asian students in clinical settings. University students, especially those for whom English is a second language, must build multi-literacy skills, particularly in English, as they pursue their degrees at English-medium institutions. Students with strong English proficiency in their fields tend to perform better academically. For veterinary medical students, the ability to handle complex tasks during clinical placements is expected. They must be able to interpret medical cases, diagnose conditions, explain treatments to clients, draft referrals and write medical reports. Mastery of English, particularly in reading, writing and speaking, is critical to understanding the specific academic language used in veterinary medicine. Language barriers can impact communication between vets and clients (Diamond et al., 2014). Those who struggle with English often face difficulties in good quality of communication (Diamond et al., 2014; Wisnivesky et al., 2019). Given the importance of English in veterinary education, this chapter highlights the language challenges faced by students at an Asian veterinary school and discusses how they should be prepared to meet the linguistic demands of their future careers. The analyses are built upon original interviews with different parties including veterinary practitioners and nurses, which suggest recommendations for educators to include in their programmes as multiple teaching tools.

An urgency: The formations of patient-centred veterinary curriculums with cultural competency training

The current communication training in veterinary schools presents a range of challenges, especially in content-heavy programmes where it is difficult to integrate communication training into the curriculum (Haldane et al., 2017). Although strong communication is essential for veterinarian practitioners, clients and patients to improve relationship, streamline clinical flows and lower staff turnover (McDermott et al., 2015), it still does not receive enough focus from veterinary educators. As a consequence, numerous studies have shown that some veterinary students and professionals lack adequate communication abilities during consultations, which perhaps prevents them from achieving certain outcomes, such as agreeing on next steps with clients or reaching a consensus on patient treatment plans (Adams & Kurtz, 2017; Bowman et al., 1992; Hamood et al., 2014; Kurtz et al., 2017). One of the common communication challenges involves handling difficult conversations or delivering bad news (Pun, 2020). Mastering the skill of communicating bad news is crucial, as a client's trust can be easily damaged in such situations. Practitioner-client relationships are especially vulnerable when conversations involve delivering bad news. Therefore, veterinarians must address their clients' emotional needs by using appropriate communication strategies to lessen negative emotions and minimise the risk of causing trauma (Clarke & Braun, 2014; Landau et al., 2015). Breaking bad news is even more challenging when veterinarians deal with vulnerable populations, such as children and the elderly (Clarke & Braun, 2014). To meet the needs of these groups, veterinarians should adjust their communication approaches accordingly. When communicating with children, it is crucial to use specific strategies to reduce the unnecessary emotional impact during their developmental stages. In cases where a pet is sick or facing death, it is advised that veterinarians first consult with the parents to determine what is the best way to convey the difficult news to the children (Clarke & Braun, 2014). A simple, honest and compassionate approach should be employed when speaking with children (Clarke & Braun, 2014). Similarly, when working with elderly clients, veterinarians should recognise the deep connection between the elderly and their pets. emphasises the importance of effective communication skills to resolve such situations without creating additional trauma to these clients (Landau et al., 2015). Veterinarians who are skilled at delivering bad news can avoid becoming defensive during difficult conversations and allow clients time to process and understand the distressing information.

Veterinarians should also assess their clients' preferences before delivering bad news. In human medicine, several communication frameworks provide structured, step-by-step approaches for this, such as the *COMFORT* (Communication, Orientation, Mindfulness, Family, Ongoing, Reiterative messages and Team) *model* (Villagran et al., 2010) and the *SPIKES protocol* (Setting, Perception, Invitation, Knowledge, Empathetic Response, Summary) (Baile et al., 2000), both of which are commonly used. However, there remains a gap in research for a communication model specifically tailored to veterinarians for breaking bad news (Pun, 2020), particularly in Asian contexts. Similar to medical doctors, veterinarians experience significant stress when delivering distressing information, adding to their occupational burden (Ballantyne & Buller, 2015). Therefore, it is crucial for veterinary educators to train veterinary students in effective communication techniques to prepare them for delivering bad news and to teach necessary strategies for reducing stress caused by miscommunication in real-life scenarios.

Linguistic and communication challenges faced by students in multilingual veterinary clinics in Hong Kong

Most undergraduate students enrolled in local veterinary programme are second-language (L2) English speakers. Upon graduation, they are expected to be proficient in both English and Cantonese in their professional roles (Pun, 2021). Throughout their studies, students have to demonstrate strong English skills to access textbooks, research articles, journals and reports, as these are predominantly published in English (Lornark & Muangsamai, 2010). However, they often lack the guidance to develop these essential skills (Elkılıç, 1994). During clinical placements, veterinary students are tasked with challenging responsibilities, including interpreting medical cases, diagnosing, explaining their recommended treatment plans and writing referrals and medical reports (Pun, 2021). To better understand the learning difficulties students face during their studies and help prepare them for the linguistic demands of their future careers, it is essential that they become proficient in English and familiar with the academic genres specific to veterinary medicine (Pun, 2021). Thus, strong

English language skills are critical for both their academic success and future careers.

The complex linguistic veterinary clinic in Hong Kong: Problems emerging from code-mixing, code-switching, translation and translanguaging

As a former British colony and now a special administrative region of China, Hong Kong has a rich cultural and linguistic landscape. The city's population is multicultural, including groups like the Japanese, Indonesians and British. Hong Kong has two official languages, Chinese (spoken as Cantonese and Putonghua, with standard written Chinese) and English. Due to the city's linguistic diversity, various multicultural speech communities have developed, fostering linguistic pluralism (Pun J., 2021). Although Cantonese is the primary language spoken by about 90 per cent of the population, this doesn't mean that most people solely communicate in Cantonese. Influenced by different speech communities and cultures, it is common in Hong Kong for individuals to engage in code-switching (alternating between two or more languages) (Hymes, 1964), code-mixing (blending two languages to create a unique code with distinct structural traits) (Maschler, 1998), translanguaging (using linguistic features from multiple languages to enhance communication) (García, 2009) and translation in both daily life and professional settings (Li, 2015).

While several studies examine veterinary practitioners' and students' perspectives on communication, culturally and linguistically competent veterinary care in Hong Kong remains limited (Englar et al., 2016; Shaw et al., 2004; Show & Englar, 2018). Deficiencies in language skills or miscommunication caused by cultural and linguistic differences can lead to misunderstandings or even legal problems (Mauranen, 2006). Despite the general consensus among veterinarians on the importance of communication for effective clinical practice, many researchers overlook the nuances of bilingual and multilingual contexts (Maschler, 1998; Englar, 2019a; 2019b), especially within a multicultural setting like Hong Kong (Pun, 2021).

First-hand thoughts from veterinary students and practitioners on teaching and communication

Pun (2021) identified three key overarching themes that emerged from the veterinary students' perceptions towards veterinary communication in the multilingual environment of Hong Kong, namely (1) gaps between teaching and real-life practising in bilingual clinical settings, (2) what constitutes effective communication in a veterinary clinic, and (3) the importance of mastering interpersonal interactive skills. The subsections below elaborate on these key aspects in detail with original transcripts.

Veterinary students' perspectives: The use of language

Educational background and language use

Before analysing the participating students' thoughts, this section offers a brief introduction of their educational background in order to facilitate the reader's understanding of their language use in school and clinical practices. A total of fifty students (first-year: n = 37, second-year: n = 13) were invited to share their perspectives on communication in their veterinary education as well as training. The participants ranged in age from 17 to 22, with 78 per cent being female and 21 per cent male. Of these, 63 per cent had completed their secondary education in Hong Kong, and 30 per cent had taken the Hong Kong Diploma of Secondary Education, the local public exam for university entry. Additionally, 10 per cent had taken the General Certificate of Education or International Baccalaureate. Half of the students had also taken the International English Language Testing System, and 5 per cent had completed the Test of English as a Foreign Language to evaluate their English skills.

In terms of linguistic backgrounds, 55 per cent of the students spoke Cantonese as their first language, and half were fluent in at least one additional language. Furthermore, 48 per cent had lived abroad for over a month in English-speaking countries such as the United States, the United Kingdom or Canada. All students self-assessed their English abilities, with 33 per cent rating themselves at the C2 level, 27 per cent at C1, 13 per cent at A2, and 7 per cent at B2 and A1.

All students in the study had received their secondary education in English, with written materials and exams primarily in that language. Of the participants, 32 per cent had English as their sole medium of instruction during secondary school. When asked about how often English was used for verbal interactions in class, the majority reported frequent use (42 per cent always, 31 per cent mostly, 21 per cent sometimes, 5 per cent rarely and 0 per cent never). In terms of their perspectives on English being the medium of instruction at university, 58 per cent believed that the English learning environment offered significant benefits, while 42 per cent felt that the advantages outweighed the drawbacks.

Everyday training vs workplace placements: The frequency of the use of the English language in veterinary educational activities

Table 9.1 shows the participating veterinary students' reported responses on the frequency of English communication in their university activities.

English was the primary written language used throughout the participating students' veterinary training. Over 85 per cent of the participants reported that formal assessments were 'always' conducted in English, both in written and spoken formats. They also mentioned that the additional reading materials provided were consistently in English. For oral communication, more than 60 per cent of students noted that regular classroom activities such as lectures, instructor feedback sessions and lab work were 'always' conducted in English, while the rest observed these activities were 'sometimes' in English. However, for student-based activities like group discussions and off-campus experiences including internships, the use of English varied significantly, ranging from

Table 9.1 Participating Veterinary Students' Reports on English Communication in University Activities

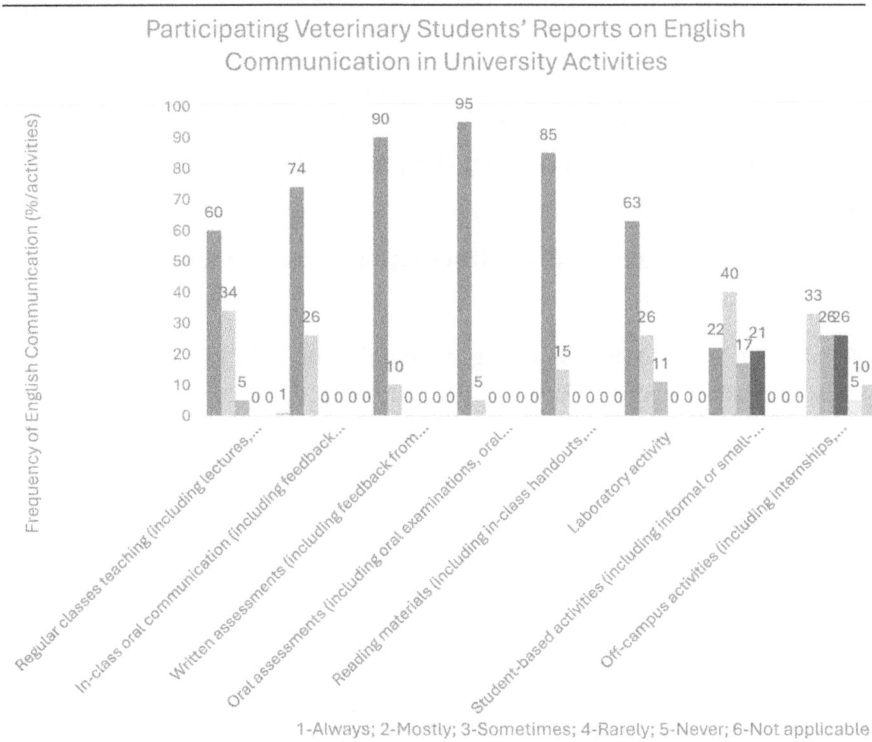

'rarely' to 'mostly'. Only 22 per cent of students 'always' communicated in English during student-led discussions, and none reported 'always' using English in off-campus activities.

Though 55 per cent of the students identified Cantonese as their first language, English was predominantly used in their veterinary education. The survey findings revealed that while English was the main language in instructor-led courses and activities, students were less likely to use it during peer-led activities, particularly in off-campus experiences like internships. This highlighted a discrepancy between the heavy reliance on English in university-based training and the more flexible use of languages in real-world clinical settings during the students' placements.

Veterinary practitioners' perceptions towards the nature of workplace communication

Pun (2021) carried out one-to-one interviews with five veterinary clinicians, respectively, which invited them to share their perceptions on bilingual workplace communication in Hong Kong. Overall, the participating clinicians agreed that they could implement effective communication by creating a mutual understanding ground with the pet owners. They further noted the significance of being competent in interpersonal communication as this could significantly foster effective interactions with pet owners and other clinicians by developing trusting clinician-client and clinician-clinician bonds.

Communicating across disciplines and interacting with pet owners effectively

Veterinarians need to develop strong communication skills to interact effectively with both clients and colleagues from various departments in the clinic. Collaboration among teams of specialists and clinicians is a common procedure when treating animals. As highlighted by a veterinary nurse in quote 1, clear communication between veterinary clinicians and their coworkers is essential to delivering quality care. Poor communication within the clinic can endanger the well-being of the pets, potentially leading to fatalities and customer complaints (Pun, 2020). One primary cause of clinical errors is the lack of communication between receptionists and veterinary surgeons (Kinnison et al., 2015). Many veterinary surgeons value their independence, but an individualistic mindset perhaps does not contribute positively to a veterinary team (Kinnison et al.,

Table 9.2 Interview Transcripts of Veterinary Clinicians' Perceptions on Clinical Communication

Role	Excerpt	Summary
Nurses	**1**	'Most of our specialists in the hospital, all of them do speak English, so usually they would communicate with each other directly . . . That is where when it comes into professional terms like they would all use the professional terminology . . . also like in different short-term like they will shorten terms a little bit because they would probably understand each other anyway because they have gone through similar training.'
	2	'To ensure that the client understands the explanation, information must follow the basic rules of communication, which are completeness, conciseness and clarity, and to also support with confirmation and documentation.'
	3	'We need to make sure the client understands what we are talking and also we act as a bridge between the company and the client. So, it's important we give clear, concise information to the clients because sometimes it's difficult for them to understand the medical terms.'
	4	'It is important to differentiate between professional language and layman's language because you don't want to be speaking professional language to the owner unless they are medical professionals . . . So you would want to be able to explain in layman's terms what the doctors actually said and what the terms actually mean so that they have a full understanding of what's going on with their pets.'
	5	'This involves choosing between open and closed questions because if we ask clients open-ended questions instead of close-ended questions we get very different answers.'
	6	'One time I had a patient coming in, and we were trying to explain the medication to the owner. And then over the conversation we found that the helper at home had been feeding the animal patient the wrong dosage of medication because she did not really understand the instruction on the label. So what we decided to do then was to have one of our Filipino colleagues in the clinic . . . helps us translate the English label into Filipino.'
	7	'So sometimes language really does become a barrier because I think Hong Kong not only speaks three languages, sometimes it is like Japanese, sometimes it's Korean . . . So when that actually comes into, when language actually comes into a problem, then we definitely would want to make sure that everyone is on the same page. For example, if they have like a pug or some really short-nose dog like brachycephalic dogs, and then they definitely want to maybe increase the size of the nostrils like how do you explain that to the owner? Is that they kind of draw a picture maybe of the nostril and then kind of this is how I am going to cut open . . . And he will kind of draw it out for you, so that's how we usually do it in a surgery setting.'

(Continued)

Table 9.2 (Continued)

Role	Excerpt	Summary
	8	'Because sometimes the owner will feel really bad or like feel really bad about making this decision and then feel like they are killing the animal. But it is actually not the case because we always tell the owner that you are actually advocating for the animal, you are actually trying to make the best decision for the animal to stop their suffering . . . So you are actually helping them to make a decision . . . as vet professionals, we all always want the best things for our animals, and then when it comes to the quality of life.'
	9	'If the client feels sad, if I told her it is better to euthanize the animals, then maybe you give a hug is a body language. Then, better than you use any words.'
	10	'I think the most important thing to bear in mind is that you always want to stand in other people is shoes when you communicate with them, no matter whether it is the doctor or it is the owner his or herself because that is how you know . . . what their concerns are and what they need.'
	11	'We need to show empathy toward clients, but we should also never obscure the facts and never mislead or give falsehoods by not communicating complete, unbiased information to the client.'
Vets	**1**	'I always ask questions in a very precise manner, so that allows the owner to tell you what you want by directing, giving them a good question, so that they can answer your question in a . . . very concise way . . . we only have 15 min in the consultation . . . So you need to re-target what you want them to say and what you want to hear.'
	2	'When you are talking to a vet over the phone, they know exactly where the lesion is and what you're talking about. There's obviously a difference when you talk to a technician because they might not necessarily have the medical background. But adjust it to the way they would understand it . . . Nurses might not have a significant scientific knowledge as your technicians or colleagues. Adjust your terminology and adjust your tone to allow them to understand and be confident and comfortable working alongside with you.'
	3	'I try to use concise sentences to summarise what has happened so that owner probably will remember the last sentence I said, which is usually the most important sentence.'
	4	'A lot of time, we have a different ethical background compared to Western countries and unfortunately, we lack this kind of background in the Western training. So, it is often very difficult, for example in the context of animal welfare, we are quite behind . . . It involves a lot of communication and thorough talking to clients to make them aware that we are not here to take away the life of your dog.'
	5	'They have a concern, there is something wrong with their pets, so it is very difficult to bring them sad news . . . That is why it is very important for us to build a relationship with our clients, so that they can trust us, and adhere to our recommendation. For example . . . I had a dog whose owner thought had a very end-stage disease as previously diagnosed by another vet. Through . . . quite a lot of communication with different owners, we then realised it was not a terminal disease. It was in fact, the beginning of a disease, which we could help and control. That is why I feel like it is very important for us to really talk to clients heart to heart,

2015). Limited time for communication often leads to disorganised team communication, thus increasing the risk of misunderstandings and medical mistakes (Pun, 2020). To avoid these issues, participating veterinary clinicians agreed that team members must communicate clearly and directly (Pun, 2021). Therefore, enhancing clinician-to-clinician communication across different specialities is an urgent priority.

Tackling confusion: The use of simple and concise wording

Given Hong Kong's cultural diversity, veterinarians face complex challenges when addressing sensitive yet common topics in veterinary medicine like the loss of a pet. According to veterinary nurses in quotes 2 and 3, clinicians had their own interpretations of what constitutes effective communication.

It is important for veterinary professionals to use straightforward language while providing detailed explanations, as this improves clients' understanding and helps clinicians gather information efficiently. As mentioned by a vet in quote 4, veterinarians can communicate in a concise manner by asking clients specific questions during the brief consultation time. Additionally, verbal communication should be supported by written communication, and vice versa, to ensure clients are well-informed during decision-making processes. Implementing mandatory verification processes, in any form, is essential to guarantee that the clients fully understand and have realistic expectations.

Code-switching between medical terms and layman languages: Know your audience

The interviewed veterinarians also shared the strategy of code-switching between medical and layman terms according to the receivers' roles and backgrounds in quotes 5 and 6. The participants indicated that they would adjust their language depending on whether they were speaking to veterinary specialists, technicians or clients with limited medical knowledge. In clinical communication, the terminology used by professionals differs significantly from everyday language. If veterinarians fail to tailor their language appropriately when speaking to clients, both Chinese-speaking and English-speaking clients with little medical background may struggle to understand. Therefore, using more accessible and everyday terms when explaining complex medical concepts is essential to ensure clients comprehend the information.

In quotes 7 and 8, the participants suggested strategies for conveying messages clearly and efficiently. For example, veterinarians would ask a mix of open-ended and closed-ended questions to gather medical information from the clients and highlight the most critical details in the final sentence to make them more memorable.

All the interviewed veterinary clinicians agreed that effective communication involves delivering information clearly, concisely and comprehensively. They also recognised the importance of switching between professional terminology and layman's language, depending on the person they are addressing.

The complex multilingual flow of veterinary communication: The problem of translanguaging

Veterinary clinicians in Hong Kong often face difficulties communicating effectively in a multicultural and multilingual environment, as the population commonly uses Cantonese, English and Mandarin (Pun, 2020). The clinicians involved highlighted the importance of not only using English but also Cantonese and Mandarin in the clinic. One veterinary doctor noted that around 90 per cent of their clients speak primarily Cantonese, which can create challenges for practitioners educated mainly in English. To address this language barrier, the participating veterinary nurses reported to have been frequently asked to serve as translators in order to facilitate communication between clients and foreign veterinarians by translating between Chinese and English. However, this translation process can complicate communication and increase the risk of misunderstandings due to potential inaccuracies, as demonstrated by Figure 9.1.

As shown in Figure 9.1, the communication process between bilingual veterinary doctors, nurses and clients is inherently complex. The sequence typically involves the following steps: (1) the client speaks to the veterinary nurse in Cantonese or Mandarin, (2) the nurse translates the client's concerns from Cantonese or Mandarin into English for the foreign veterinarian, (3) the veterinarian records the consultation details, including the pet's medical history, examinations and diagnosis, in written medical English, (4) the veterinarian conducts a physical examination using non-verbal communication, and (5) both the veterinarian and nurse communicate the pet's diagnosis and suggest a treatment plan to the client.

Due to the multilingual environment in Hong Kong, veterinary clinicians frequently encounter communication challenges, as they often need to assist clients who are not fluent in English. One participant described in quote 9 an

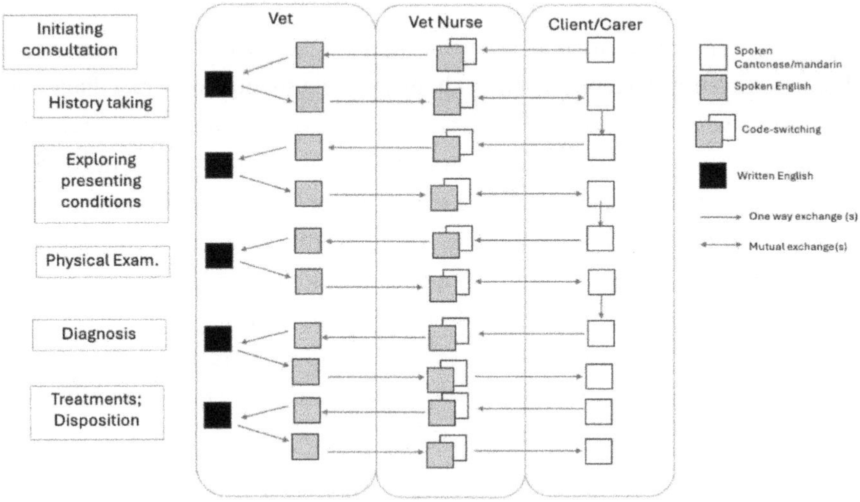

Figure 9.1 Bilingual flow communication chart in veterinary practices

incident where a Filipino helper misunderstood the pet's medication dosage. Besides translation issues, a nurse mentioned in quote 10 that communication difficulties could also arise when explaining treatments and procedures to clients with limited language proficiency.

Cultural clashes on animal welfare

In addition to language issues, the participating clinicians also noted that Hong Kong's cultural landscape makes veterinary communication in local settings quite distinct from that in other cultures, particularly Western ones. Cultural differences can sometimes lead to misunderstandings, especially on sensitive topics such as euthanasia. Therefore, it is crucial for veterinary practitioners and nurses to clearly provide clients with all relevant animal welfare information, ensuring clients are well-informed and respected in their decisions, regardless of the choices they make. In quotes 11 and 12, a practitioner and nurse expressed differing ethical views, which stemmed from their contrasting cultural backgrounds.

Interpersonal communication: Gathering patients' medical histories, diagnosing conditions and delivering difficult news

Extending on the cultural aspects, the participating veterinarians stressed the importance of developing interpersonal communication skills. They highlighted the need to show empathy and build rapport with clients to foster honest interactions. By adopting a relationship-focused approach, veterinarians can obtain more truthful responses from clients, leading to more accurate diagnoses and improved treatment plans for pets, as discussed in quote 13. This becomes especially critical when delivering difficult news or ensuring clients adhere to recommended treatments. Despite the importance of establishing trust, misunderstandings can arise from how clients' questions are perceived. For instance, one practitioner viewed frequent questioning as a sign of mistrust, while a nurse saw it as an indicator of a strong relationship.

Veterinary practitioners and nurses can also demonstrate compassion and empathy by offering emotional support like comforting a client with a hug. In quotes 14 and 15, the nurses emphasised the importance of putting themselves in the clients' position, which fosters better communication and helps them better understand clients' concerns and needs.

The interviewees also mentioned the need for patience, allowing clients time to process distressing news about their pets before pushing them to make decisions. However, the interviewees stressed in quote 16 that empathy should be expressed genuinely, without creating false expectations or misunderstandings for the clients.

How to adjust the veterinary curriculum to train students for bilingual clinical contexts?

This chapter compares the perspectives of veterinary medical students and clinicians on communication requirements in Hong Kong's bilingual environment. As the findings showed, English plays a critical role in veterinary communication, with both groups agreeing that it is widely used in the field. Over half of the students saw the use of English as the primary medium of instruction as a major advantage, highlighting the language's importance in both academic and clinical settings.

Although veterinary students receive their education primarily in English, many programmes do not address the communication challenges that arise from language differences between veterinarians and clients (Landau et al., 2015). Language barriers can negatively affect healthcare services, including veterinary care (Irvine et al., 2006). In Hong Kong, veterinarians often communicate medical instructions in either English, Cantonese or Mandarin, depending on the client or colleague. Miscommunication between veterinarians and non-English or Cantonese-speaking clients can lead to medical errors such as improper medication use. According to the study, a gap exists between students' language use in university and that in clinical practice. While English is essential in both veterinary schools and clinics, other languages, such as Cantonese and Mandarin, are frequently spoken in clinics. Students noted that they often used languages other than English during internships and work placements, revealing an inconsistency between their educational experience and the realities of the workplace. This finding further underscored the need to consider cultural factors when teaching veterinary communication.

The participating clinicians also emphasised the importance of switching between professional and everyday language accordingly. Both students and recent graduates can find it challenging to navigate this shift (Dahm, 2011). According to Dahm (2012), clinicians should avoid using medical jargon when speaking with clients, as medical terminology can be understood differently by the two parties. Explaining complex concepts in simpler terms helps veterinarians communicate more effectively with clients of varying educational backgrounds. In Hong Kong, veterinarians must be confident in communicating in English, Cantonese and Mandarin, as well as using layman's language. Mastering both medical and everyday language in a bilingual setting is already difficult (Bourhis et al., 1989), and it becomes even more challenging when this needs to be done in three languages (Pun, 2021). Therefore, veterinary schools should offer bilingual or trilingual training environments to fully equip students with the necessary communication skills for clinical practice. Additionally, communication training should include the cultural dimensions of Hong Kong. According to a pair of participating nurse and vet, locals and Westerners in Hong Kong hold different views on animal welfare. Veterinary students must be equipped to handle sensitive issues like euthanasia, as it is not enough to rely on the Western model of veterinary education, which may overlook important cultural differences and hinder communication.

The participating veterinary clinicians also stressed that effective clinical communication requires clear, complete and concise interactions. While veterinary communication has many unique aspects (Kinnison et al., 2015), interpersonal communication skills are often seen as equally important as language proficiency. Thus, veterinary schools should provide students with comprehensive communication training. One of the main goals of medical training programmes, in general, has always been to enhance communication skills (Waitzkin, 1984). By showing empathy, engaging in honest discussions and providing emotional support, veterinarians can build trust and rapport with clients (Pun, 2021). To help students develop these skills, educators often use techniques like role-playing, simulations and working with standardised clients (Radford et al., 2003; Mclaughlin et al., 2008; Nogueira et al., 2008; Whelan et al., 2005). These methods help students discover their strengths as communicators, understand their clients' needs and identify areas for improvement in veterinary practice (Mclaughlin et al., 2008; Nogueira et al., 2008).

Limitations: A tendency to generalise clinicians' perceptions and research gap in multilingual veterinary communication

This study, while offering valuable insights into veterinary communication in Hong Kong's bilingual context, had certain limitations. Since only one local university provides a veterinary medicine programme, the pool of veterinary students available for the survey was quite small, resulting in a limited sample size for the quantitative questionnaires. Additionally, there has been little research on veterinary communication in bilingual or multilingual environments. Although this lack of prior studies makes establishing a foundation for current research more challenging, it also points to research gaps and presents opportunities for further exploration. Future studies could expand on this topic by using a larger sample size and perhaps even including the perspectives of veterinary clients to better understand their communication needs. The findings of this study suggested a potential mismatch between the language training veterinary students receive in university and the language demands they face in clinical practice.

*

To conclude, this chapter has offered original insights for researchers and veterinarians into the communication needs and perspectives of veterinary students and clinicians. The research team identified three key themes: (1) the gap between veterinary school training and real-life bilingual clinical environments in Hong Kong, (2) strategies for effective communication in clinical settings and (3) the importance of interpersonal skills. Although English is regarded as an important language by veterinary students and professionals, the study highlighted a gap between the language used in instruction and the practical demands of bilingual clinical interactions in Hong Kong. The findings emphasised the necessity of being able to communicate with clients in both languages to be an effective veterinarian in the city.

This chapter's exploration of veterinarians' perspectives can serve as a guide for educators to develop multimodal teaching resources that address the communication challenges students face in bilingual environments. These future learning tools should encourage critical reflection on communication practices in both educational and clinical contexts. Overall, the findings stress the need for a culturally adapted communication training model in Hong Kong's veterinary education. Such a model would help students develop the skills necessary to provide high-quality care to both clients and their pets. Instead of relying solely on widely used Western models, it is essential for veterinary curricula to focus on culturally appropriate communication methods, preparing students for the bilingual realities of veterinary practice in Hong Kong (Pun, 2021). Ultimately, this culturally tailored approach would improve client satisfaction and enhance the quality of care provided to pets.

While this chapter has examined communication within veterinary practice, similar challenges exist in high-risk medical settings, such as intensive care units and emergency departments. The next chapter shifts focus to critical care medicine, exploring the complexities of clinician-patient communication in high-stress environments, the importance of speaking up for patient safety and the linguistic challenges faced by medical professionals in Hong Kong's trilingual healthcare system.

Part II

Skills for effective clinical communication

10

Critical care medicine

This chapter explores the complexities of clinical communication in high-risk medical settings, focusing on Intensive Care Units (ICUs) and Emergency Departments (EDs) in Hong Kong. Drawing on three empirical studies, it examines the perspectives of ICU clinicians, mechanically ventilated (MV) patients, and ED clinicians within a multilingual and multicultural Chinese context. The chapter first investigates the concept of communication openness among ICU doctors and nurses, highlighting the role of psychological safety, hierarchical dynamics, and language strategies in shaping clinicians' willingness to speak up. It also addresses the often-overlooked communication needs of conscious MV patients, whose intended messages span beyond task-related content to include emotional, medical, and personal domains. The chapter then turns to the ED context, identifying major communication challenges such as code-switching, inconsistent documentation, and miscommunication during handovers and triage. It concludes by proposing targeted strategies—such as structured communication training, inclusive leadership practices, and culturally sensitive tools—to enhance clinician-patient interactions, shared decision-making, and team communication in critical care environments.

Why is communication in high-risk settings important?

To make accurate diagnoses and plan suitable medical treatments, clinical communication plays a key element worldwide. In an interpersonal aspect, effective healthcare interactions aid patients in understanding relevant medical information and thereby facilitate their medical care by building trust and making them feel satisfied (Health Canada, 2004). As per various global studies, insufficient and inaccurate clinical communication puts patient safety at risk, especially in high-risk settings like Intensive Care Units (ICUs) and Emergency Departments (EDs) (Lingard et al., 2004; Sutcliffe et al., 2004; Apker et al., 2007; Kachalia et al., 2007; Cheung et al., 2010; Slade et al., 2015). From these studies, we can understand that patients' experiences of critical scenarios including severe diseases and deaths as well as the compromise of the quality of medical services (e.g. delayed deliveries of healthcare, inaccurate diagnoses, unsuitable medical treatments) may occur when communication in high-risk settings is ineffective (Chisholm et al., 2000; Coiera et al., 2002; Ye et al., 2007; Cheung et al., 2010; Evans, 2015).

Observing these issues, this chapter reviews three studies in Hong Kong that include interviews with ICU clinicians, mechanically ventilated (MV) patients and ED clinicians to explore more comprehensive perspectives from different parties in a multicultural and multilingual Asian context. This chapter first explores ICU doctors' and nurses' perceptions of communication openness perceptions in a Hong Kong hospital and states the communication challenges they face. By researching their communication within the ICU and across departments, this chapter illustrates why they speak up and how to encourage them to do so. The chapter then moves on to address a knowledge gap in the interactive needs of MV patients who are conscious but incapable of verbally articulating themselves. Including pieces of interview transcripts (interviews were conducted using the stimulated recall technique) with ten recovered patients who were formerly MV in a multidisciplinary ICU for at least 24 hours before the occurrences of interviews. This chapter demonstrates the multidimensional intended scope of communication content of MV patients beyond task-focused topics (Leung et al., 2018), including (1) medical discussions with their doctors and nurses; (2) interactions with family members to give advice as well as comfort; (3) stating their requests and plans; (4) expressing their feelings and letting others know their personal perspectives on treatments; and (5) conveying their psycho-emotional needs.

This chapter also includes a study of a Hong Kong ED to expand the scope of clinical communication in Asian high-risk settings. The last section focuses on the unique context of Hong Kong EDs and relevant communication problems, which reflects on the complexity of trilingual healthcare communication in Hong Kong. The findings were generated from twenty-eight interviews with key ED doctors and nurses, which presented linguistic evidence related to shared decision-making processes and communication challenges clinicians face during trilingual clinical interactions in a multicultural Chinese context.

Why should clinicians speak up in high-risk clinical contexts?

According to Ayoko (2007), the term communication openness means the state of people being at ease when interacting with one another verbally and the extent to which they acquire understanding when conversing. Ever since, this term has been used with trust, listening, honesty as well as support. Based on Ayoko's (2007) definition of the term, Rogers et al. (2007) noted that communication openness concerns behaviours that are associated with sending and receiving messages among different parties like superiors, subordinates and peers. Applying this term in the context of medical interactions, Nolan (2000) indicated that it is essential to lower the risks to patient safety as clinicians feel safe and able to speak up freely. Poor communication and teamwork failure can risk patient safety (Leonard et al., 2004). Lyndon et al. (2012) and Schwappach and Gehring (2014) explained that 'speaking up' is an action for medics to talk about their concerns regarding patient safety by asking immediate questions and/or articulating their opinions or information until they come up with a clear resolution is found and when their seniors omit messages or make mistakes (Entwistle et al., 2010). Unfortunately, a lot of healthcare workers, junior ones in particular, have a tendency to keep silent and are hesitant to speak up even when patient safety is at risk due to medical errors (Morrison & Milliken, 2003). To ensure that there are no medical errors and eliminate potential risks to patient safety, it is crucial for medics to be able to speak up about their concerns. To achieve so, hospitals should ensure their clinicians' psychological safety, which means clinicians should feel that they can voice their ideas, ask questions, raise concerns or point out errors without fear of humiliation, shame, or guilt and that they can talk about their thoughts and feelings and take risks (Eppich, 2015; Edmondson, 2012, 1999). Any disruptive behaviours in high-risk healthcare settings can threaten clinicians' safety. These include raising one's voice and expressing a condescending attitude to each other or junior medics (Eppich, 2015). Some clinicians are afraid of speaking up because they fear that their concerns will be considered signs of ignorance, incompetency, negativity and even disruptive behaviours by their colleagues (Eppich, 2015; Edmondson, 2012).

To learn about to what extent clinicians feel safe to speak up for their patients' benefit, researchers often look at their levels of communication openness. Individual and contextual factors greatly influence clinicians' willingness and motivations to speak up accordingly. A lot of clinicians find that the hierarchy of a hospital and interdisciplinary practices avoids them from speaking up

(Schwappach & Gehring, 2014). Carter et al.'s (2013) study found that British clinicians deemed it inappropriate for them to speak up to their seniors and negative consequences would arise, including positive relationships falling apart. The factors that affect clinicians' perceptions regarding the pros and cons of speaking up are individual such as tenure, work, e.g. work configuration, organisational context including culture, data like benchmarking as well as the external environment such as attention. Luong et al. (2009) further discovered that nurses and managers from traditional Asian family backgrounds tend to be less willing to speak up. As for the unique context of Hong Kong, Law and Chan (2015) found that nurses lack understanding and trust across generations and that senior clinicians seldom listen to nursing students' motivation to speak up for patient safety. Therefore, cultural factors are often a barrier to speaking up, especially in Chinese healthcare settings.

Do ICU clinicians in Hong Kong feel safe enough to speak up?

Ng et al.'s (2017a) study of the speak-up culture in a Hong Kong ICU showed that while the participating ICU clinicians seemed to have a similar perception of their levels of communication openness with their colleagues, doctors tended to have a more positive attitude regarding communication openness than their nursing colleagues in a number of aspects. However, the participating nurses showed a slightly more positive attitude towards nursing leadership, doctor leadership and the understanding of patient-care goals. The participating ICU doctors and nurses also had different perceptions of the speak-up culture within the unit. The primary reasons for them to speak up were usually looking for information and clarification. Some other factors also affected their motivations to speak up as well as relevant practices, including ranks, language and communication training. To ensure that ICU clinicians are able to speak up freely, hospitals should create a safe space that advocates the value of equal status among colleagues. This allows clinicians to be confident enough to talk to each other openly and discuss their personal thoughts without fearing reprisal or experiencing embarrassment.

Speaking up across ranks, communication timeliness, understanding of patient care aims, leadership and overall effectiveness

Ng et al. (2017) explored ICU clinicians' thoughts about the level of satisfaction regarding communication and teamwork within the unit and illustrated their thoughts about communication openness. These aspects were highlighted: (1) clinician-clinician interactions across different ranks and departments, (2) communicating timely, (3) clinicians' understanding of patient-care goals, (4) the effectiveness of leadership within the team and (5) the overall effectiveness of the unit.

1. The participants generally demonstrated a positive evaluation of workplace communication. The highest levels of satisfaction were found in communication between senior doctors and from senior doctors to their colleagues from other ranks and departments. The participating nurses had a lower level of satisfaction regarding their communication with other colleagues.
2. The participating clinicians were highly satisfied with communication timeliness as in passing on information related to patient care. However, the nurses had a lower level of satisfaction than the doctors.
3. The clinicians in general had a slightly positive attitude towards the extent to which they understand patient care goals, including patient care plans, their respective duties when executing the care plans, and the potential threats to patient safety.
4. When compared to their levels of satisfaction with the other aspects, the participants were slightly less satisfied with the leadership in the ICU.
5. They also found that the effectiveness within the unit was ideal.

Ng et al. (2017) also noted that there were minor positive correlations between ICU staff who had previously received communication training and their ability to communicate openly and understand patient-care goals. Therefore, it is important for ICU clinicians to receive sufficient communication training as it can improve their self-reported ability to speak up openly and understand patient-care goals.

How to motivate clinicians to speak up? What makes them speak up?

In Ng et al.'s (2017) study, the participating senior ICU nurses stated that they would speak up when it concerned issues about patient transfer, nursing handovers and patient follow-up related to their treatments and medications. By speaking up, they could ensure that the transfer of information was effective for their patients' benefit. One of them said that they would use the strategy of repeating information they received until they were sure that both they and their colleagues had a full understanding of the piece of information.

> *[Nurses] might request additional information or ask for information to be clarified when information was lacking or unclear in the handover documents.*
>
> *[We would speak up] when we felt that we needed to know more about a case for effective follow-up or to clarify the current stage reached in the prescribed clinical treatment for the patient.*

For the participating doctors, they would mostly speak in the situation in which they acquired more information and had to clarify messages, especially during handovers and shift changes as well as the decision-making processes that concerned their patients' treatments. Speaking up allowed them to continue treatments smoothly and have the information needed for decision-making processes relevant to treatments. Therefore, both ICU doctors' and nurses' most common reasons for speaking up were seeking or clarifying information. Nearly none of them would speak up within the unit due to 'classic' reasons like pointing out mistakes (e.g. potentially inaccurate diagnoses, inappropriate medical treatments) and any rule violations or failure to work based on standardised procedures.

What encourages them to speak up and how to help them?

All of the interviewed ICU doctors and nurses in Ng et al.'s (2017) study found the unit capable of encouraging them to speak up when needed, which might be related to their proclivity for implementing speak-up practices. They similarly shared a view towards the elements that would advocate the speak-up culture within the unit:

1. Their familiarity with the ICU patients' information and conditions in the ICU affects their willingness to speak up.
2. They felt safer speaking up if there were no apparent hierarchies within the unit and if they had more chances to express their views regardless of their ranks and specialities.
3. They would want to have more opportunities to ask questions and be part of medical discussions, which could be achieved if relationship conflicts between them and their colleagues across ranks were reduced. Trusting relationships could be built if everyone in the team could be respectful of

each other, especially those who were familiar with a patient's case and willing to discuss any relevant concerns.

Hierarchies and conflicts were some key factors that created tension and communication barriers within the team, which made them uncertain about speaking up for patient safety. Some of the participating nurses shared that the major factor that motivated them to speak up in critical situations was to be regarded as someone with an equal professional status without the hindrance of the hierarchical structure within the unit:

A senior nurse commented, 'We should listen to staff who spend the most time by the bedside of the patients, as nurses will clearly know the clinical development of the patients.'

Training sessions

As noted, training sessions are a useful tool for the promotion of the culture of speaking up in the ICU. A lot of the participants in Ng et al.'s (2017) study were not aware of the communication training sessions offered by the Hospital Authority that aimed to guide them to speak up. Clinicians who had received training on crew resource management (CRM) added that existing training programmes usually focused on merely team dynamics and effective leadership in critical situations. However, they noted that there was a lack of courses that were helpful to the facilitation of clinician-clinician communication during daily routine duties.

Learning to speak up across ranks and with other departments

As noted, hierarchies are often a hindrance to clinicians' speak-up practices worldwide. Ng et al.'s (2017) study found that it was the case for ICU clinicians in Hong Kong as well. The participating nursing staff shared in the interviews that they were only willing to speak up to doctors when it was absolutely essential for them to follow up on patient cases, patients' treatments and medications. The nurses were also more likely to speak up than the doctors. These nurses also tended to just comply with the doctors' instructions. The participating ICU doctors would also only talk to the nurses if they needed help with very urgent cases. Moreover, the nurses often had very limited time to interact with the doctors as the doctors tended to be very busy with their duties. As a result, the participating ICU nurses would normally try to solve problems by asking for advice from the head nurse or requesting the nurse-in-charge to follow up on their questions with the corresponding doctor.

Interdisciplinary communication was another identified key factor that affected patient safety and the effectiveness of the whole unit in general. The participating clinicians found it essential for them to interact with other external disciplines including the ED and medical and surgical departments when treating patients. When doing so, the participating ICU doctors were required to confirm certain medical information with their colleagues from other departments, for instance, they had to check the medication for their patients. Unfortunately, the participants found the speak-up culture across disciplines rather underdeveloped. A lot of participating junior doctors found it difficult to talk to colleagues from other departments about patient management. They believed that they had less authority in decision-making processes when planning patient care. They noted a hierarchy in interdisciplinary interactions, for example, they were asked to just talk to other colleagues of similar ranks or levels of work experience through the telephone. They explained that it was usually deemed inappropriate for juniors to reach out to seniors from other departments directly.

To tackle communication barriers, the interviewed ICU doctors and nurses found it necessary for all clinicians to be more patient with and respectful of each other, including junior colleagues who actually were more experienced in their specialities, especially when treating patients who were not of their specialities. The interviewees stressed the importance of listening to and making an effort to understand other clinicians' thoughts. They also found it useful to encourage those who were more experienced in their specialities to speak up and share their experiences, as well as being mentors to junior colleagues.

The participants further offered some insights into various approaches to their speak-up practices across different ranks, within the unit and across disciplines. They shared their experiences regarding how junior clinicians could speak up to their seniors skilfully:

> *Junior doctors will speak up only when they have a strong, justified opinion or to clarify information related to patient harm. Senior doctors will speak up during a handover when they have more perceived role space through an understanding of their role contribution in providing a different opinion within a joint-team collaborative decision.*

Some other interviewees thought that senior doctors often had more space to express their thoughts during decision-making processes regarding patient-care plans because they had more authority. However, an interviewed senior doctor also acknowledged the need to advocate the culture of speaking up within the unit as seniors could make mistakes too.

The interviewed senior nurses observed that their juniors were quite passive when they had to ask questions during handovers. They said they were happy to open up spaces for their junior colleagues to clarify information or guide them through the process of understanding unfamiliar situations. Normally, junior nurses who had less than a year of working experience need time to learn medical jargon spoken exclusively within the unit, get familiarised with handover practices and be aware of potential risks to patient safety (Ng et al., 2017). Therefore, the interviewed senior nurses said it was important to the junior nurses to ask questions during handovers if they found the information ambiguous.

Language strategies

The interviewed ICU nurses and doctors in Ng et al.'s (2017) study adopted different language strategies when speaking up. The nurses observed that a lot of the ICU staff would neglect the significance of language use because they tended to prioritise medical issues. They agreed that one's speak-up practices depended on their individual way of speaking. Therefore, a lot of them were unaware of any particular expressions for speaking up. A senior nurse was concerned with such a situation and stressed the importance of speaking with a non-threatening tone of voice in order to make each other more comfortable when dealing with critical situations.

Some interviewed doctors also suggested that they would formulate the moment of speaking up by making factual descriptions based on their observations. They also found it crucial to offer sufficient background information before making their arguments and then allow others to assess each other's arguments. This suggested approach aligns with the steps of a medical handover designed under the systematic framework of ISBAR (Introduction, patient Situation, Background, Assessment and Recommendation of plan), which is promoted in both local and overseas hospitals (Thompson et al., 2011). The participating doctors further found open-ended questions quite useful when speaking up to make enquiries. This way, clinicians could avoid forming a judgement or jumping to conclusions and making direct decisions. Instead, the whole ICU team had the chance to express their views. Non-verbal language was also suggested, for example, they would make eye contact to signal the need to ask questions in order to encourage their junior colleagues to speak up.

The participating junior ICU doctors also found indirect communication strategies particularly useful. Instead of speaking up to senior clinicians directly, they would reach out to the whole team to assist them in reviewing lab reports and clinical images such as X-rays, which could alert senior doctors about any omitted medical information.

These suggested indirect communication strategies align with the Chinese cultural value of upholding harmony, which opens up the space for clinicians to negotiate the boundaries of role relationships flexibly without threatening others' faces or status (Pun J., 2018).

Advocating the speak-up culture in Chinese medical settings

To promote the speak-up culture in Chinese medical settings, the participating ICU clinicians in Ng et al.'s (2017) study also made the following advice:

1. Being sincere when speaking up to clinicians of different ranks or years of experience.
2. Negotiating a mutual understanding of all the latest medical information about patients in order to ensure the understanding of the members involved in decision-making processes. All messages should also be relayed with clarity, so everyone could easily digest them and make discussions accordingly.
3. Sharing a mutual speak-up language within the same unit.
4. Promoting speak-up practices between junior and senior clinicians.
5. Creating a non-blaming culture, so junior doctors would feel safe enough to speak up. The culture of reprisal should be discouraged as it would prevent the juniors from speaking up about minor problems.
6. Avoiding certain ICU colloquial expressions with varying connotations used in only one hospital.

What about the patients? Do clinicians understand the needs of what mechanically ventilated patients want to say?

Clinicians aside, MV patients in high-risk settings also often experience communication barriers. While the use of tracheal intubation and mechanical ventilation (MV) is essential for a lot of ICU patients, these patients have difficulty verbally expressing themselves under MV. When a patient requires the use of MV, they are usually suffering from critical conditions. Therefore, there is a need for them to be able to communicate and they experience frustrations when not being heard. Taking the latest medical trend of targeting light sedation or daily interruption in sedation into consideration, it is quite likely for ICU patients to suffer from long periods of time in which they are conscious but unable to speak (Kress et al., 2000; Mehta et al., 2018). Khalaila et al.'s (2011) study found that 40–80 per cent of invasively ventilated ICU patients found communication moderately to extremely difficult, and 60 per cent of the participants felt extremely frustrated with their communication needs not being met (Patak et al., 2004; Happ et al., 2011).

Existing studies have shown that conventional patient-clinician and patient-family communication during MV is regarded highly important yet of low quality for all parties involved (Leathart, 1994; Institute of Medicine Committee, 2001Happ et al., 2004; Myhren et al., 2009; Ashworth, 1980; Menzel, 1998; Broyles et al., 2012; Carroll, 2004; Tembo et al., 2015). ICU clinicians would intentionally prioritise subject matters they found crucial, including physical symptoms and care-related duties (Happ et al., 2004; Ashworth, 1980). Therefore, MV patients' needs remain neglected and misunderstandings may arise. Patients are often made to simplify their messages due to such a communication barrier (Carroll, 2004). Their physical incapability to speak effectively makes them feel distressed, anxious, angry, fear, losing control, imprisoned, depersonalised and socially isolated. It may even lead to long-term sequelae such as post-intensive care anxiety or depression (Khalaila et al., 2011; Patak et al., 2004; Happ et al., 2011; Myhren et al., 2009; Tembo et al., 2015; Carroll, 2007; Bergbom-Engberg, 1989).

The scope of communication needs of MV patients

Leung et al. (2018) employed the stimulated recall technique and carried out interviews with MV patients, which explored the intended scope of communication content of these patients. The team noted that the scope was primarily multidimensional, which included domains of medical discussions with their clinicians, and the desire to express their sense of suffering, feelings and emotions, asking for support, wanting to make plans and conveying personal perspective to their families. These communication needs were potentially unmet. Therefore, it is significant to offer ICU strategies to aid MV patients in participating in conversations about medical, non-medical and psycho-emotional topics instead of just communicating about simple symptoms or task-related matters.

The participating patients said that they wanted to engage in conversations with their clinicians as well as medical discussions actively. While some of the intended messages were about physical discomforts and were thereby simpler and more intuitive to the clinicians, others were more complex. There were some instances in which the participants wanted to express their personal perspectives about treatment-related decisions. They also wished to express their desire to limit therapy. No matter their views, ranging from reflecting their opinions to transient emotional responses, Leung et al.'s (2018) found that ICU clinicians should have a high awareness of their MV patients' feelings and thus address these issues accordingly.

The participating MV patients also added that they wanted to discuss their thoughts about their conditions with family members and connect with them as well as their friends. Therefore, they would like to be able to exchange advice, feel supported and express emotions such as love, gratitude and regret.

Skills to involve MV patients in active conversations about medical, non-medical and psycho-emotional matters

Leung et al. (2018) discovered a range of communication tools and strategies ICU clinicians used with their MV patients in Hong Kong. The researchers categorised certain widely used approaches into two aspects: (1) natural methods including the mouthing of words, nodding, facial expression and body language and (2) augmented alternative communication tools including writing, typing, alphabet boards, communication boards or other advanced electronic applications. While natural methods are easy to perform, they cannot be used to convey complex content. MV patients and their family caregivers tend to feel frustrated and have difficulties communicating using natural methods (Slade et al., 2015a).

By designing pre-determined lists of communication content, MV patients can touch/point to select what they are trying to convey. Communication boards available in Hong Kong include those offered by the Hong Kong Society of Critical Care or Vidatak EZ Board. Tablet-based digital communication applications like the Society of Critical Care Medicine's 'ICU Patient Communicator' also help them communicate easily (Hong Kong Society of Critical Care Medicine's ICU Communication Board in

Traditional Chinese, 2010; Society of Critical Care Medicine, 2001; ten Hoorn et al., 2016; Patak et al., 2006). Leung et al. (2018) identified the categories of the content included in these communication tools, including firstly, descriptions of patients' physical feelings or short expressions of feelings like 'sad'. To facilitate MV patients in describing their physical sense of discomfort such as pain in greater detail, these tools usually offer a diagram of the human body accompanied by a scale that lets them point at the locations of pain and severity. Secondly, these boards also include the phrase 'I want' that is followed by requests for various physical tasks or changes in the surrounding environments like turning the lights off. Thirdly, there are 'I want to see' signs followed by a range of options of people like doctors, nurses and family members. Fourthly, there are some pre-determined questions such as 'how am I doing?' and 'What has happened?' Finally, there is a display of alphabets and numbers that allows patients to create combinations of free text. However, while these tools are useful in helping patients in carrying out simple communications, there is still a need for expansion in order to cover sufficient communication content and thus carry out complex medical conversations between ICU clinicians, MV patients and their families regarding topics that involve offering advice, discussing feelings, thoughts and emotions (Broyles et al., 2012). The existing methods of communication through typing, writing and pointing to alphabet boards are limited to broad communication. Considering MV patients tend to be weak, have unable symptoms, suffer from oedema and have very limited mobility, vision or legibility of handwriting and literacy, the current tools are not too effective and realistically feasible.

MV patients often experience psycho-emotional issues during their non-vocal periods. The participants in Leung et al.'s (2018) recalled that they felt lonely and wanted to cry when hearing about the possibility of death from their clinicians. Other studies noted very similar findings (Khalaila et al., 2011; Patak et al., 2004; Happ et al., 2011; Tembo et al., 2015). To design effective communication tools for ICU clinicians and MV patients' family members to mitigate the patients' psycho-emotional sufferings, the first stage is to acknowledge the patients' feelings.

Challenges faced by ED clinicians in Hong Kong medical contexts

Errors in translations

Similar to other EDs in various Asian and European regions, those in Hong Kong are essentially multilingual. In local EDs, Cantonese, Mandarin and

English are spoken and written. These contexts involve the switch between these three languages because the ED clinicians' native language is mostly Chinese and they would converse bilingually or even trilingually when carrying out everyday responsibilities. Such uses of language reflect the use of local official languages and the use of the English language in tertiary teaching (Chandler et al., 2015). In actual practice, ED clinicians read and note medical information in English virtually while speaking to their patients in their native tongues. When carrying out clinician-clinician interactions, they speak to each other mostly in Cantonese mixed with English medical jargon (Slade et al., 2015a; 2015b), which is nothing like daily English and sometimes leads to discrepancies in medical documents. As a result, several times of translating processes occur during a single patient journey (Matthiessen, 2013). Additionally, clinicians' language use of code-switching makes it difficult for their patients to comprehend all languages spoken by them (Slade et al., 2016). The complex environment of trilingual space in Hong Kong and time pressures make medical documentation challenging and often lead to errors (Pun et al., 2015). In general, communication in local EDs is often at risk.Pun et al. (2015) interviewed ED clinicians in Hong Kong and identified handovers as the step in which miscommunication happened the most. The interviewed ED clinicians said it was common for doctors to give inaccurate verbal instructions and for nurses to misunderstand the sorts of medications with similar English pronunciations. One of the senior ED doctors described the impacts of communication problems that risked patients' safety:

> *Sometimes the [doctors] may give a verbal order . . . and maybe what the doctors ordered was not well-perceived by our staff. . .. And so it may lead to some misunderstanding in delivering – I mean a wrong dosage or wrong rate of infusions for the patient. And so this is one of the communication problems that I've observed . . . in the past 12 months.* (INT_Doc_1)

Another senior ED doctor explained that the process of making English medical notes was usually selective, which condensed what their patients articulated said in Cantonese:

> *Of course we have to condense a very long story into [something] concise. Because we just can't copy what the patients say. Even if they speak in English, we can't copy what they say.* (INT_Doc_5)

As for the process of explaining medical knowledge to patients, a doctor observed that communication issues would arise when they tried to translate on the spot from written English to spoken Cantonese:

> *For some specific disease that we know in English, sometimes for some rare diseases it may be difficult for us to find the right Chinese term to explain to the patient.* (INT_Doc_2)

An interviewed senior doctor recognised the fact that translations often led to omissions in or changes of medical information, and stated how they and their colleagues would solve the issue:

> *Because we have [been] doing this for so many years, we try to closely relate those Cantonese things into the notes. But sometimes actually the Cantonese cannot be directly translated into the English. I think many colleagues will put the Chinese character inside the notes.* (INT_Doc_1)

The above interview extracts illustrated the trilingual nature of local EDs and code-switch practices and thus indicated the frequency of communication barriers that emerged from these practices. Besides, the forms and errors of written medical notes are also being raised by the clinicians in the ED context. Nearly half of the interviewees in Pun et al.'s (2015) study had communication issues when making medical documentation in written forms. They shared that each colleague had their own personal preferences about what medium to use for communicating information, including written, verbal or both. Therefore, they found it unpredictable regarding how their colleagues would want to communicate and when the medium would shift. Consequently, the interviewees had to rely on their own experiences in order to understand the spoken or written details about their patients' medical history and symptoms during medical handovers as the documenting process was inconsistent. One of them said that ED communication was just like 'chaotic traffic', particularly during handovers. Clinicians might possibly omit and change relevant information.

Communication issues at triage due to time limitations and insufficient manpower

A lot of the interviewed ED clinicians in Pun et al.'s (2015) study found it the most challenging for them to communicate with each other and their patients during the key points of transitions within patients' journeys. A senior doctor discussed the situation of the triage station:

> *I think the triage is the most high-pressure area in our department because the volume of [patients] is so . . . high. Sometimes there may be 30, 40, 60 patients waiting outside in the waiting hall to be seen by the doctor, so triage became a*

> *very convenient point for them to go to the triage nurse and ask 'What's happening here? And why am I waiting here so long?' And so I think problems can arise easily in the triage area, and communication is a very important tool to overcome those problems.* (INT_Doc_2)

Unlike most other EDs, EDs in Hong Kong label triage categories explicitly to admitted patients. However, patients would still have to wait for a long time to be attended to and often experience a lack of explanations from their clinicians., which makes them frustrated. Sometimes, serious issues arise when a patient is not assigned to an appropriate triage category. A senior doctor said that dire consequences such as exacerbation or death happen when a patient was categorised in a category too low for their condition:

> *We had a patient who was referred from a GP because of leg swelling. Actually, the GP had written in the referral notes that a clot inside the blood vessel was suspected. But it was inappropriately triaged and the patient was left waiting for two hours; and then the patient collapsed and finally died of lung-primary embolism.* (INT_Doc_3)

With effective interactions, this particular tragic incident could have been prevented. Unfortunately, the responsible clinicians were not aware of the issue at triage. The interviewed doctor went on to elaborate that this patient was inaccurately triaged because of ineffective communication:

> *In terms of communication, maybe you are worried that [the triage staff] did not read the GP's letter carefully. We're not sure whether it was due to the time limitations or whether it was due to a lack of knowledge of this disease.* (INT_Doc_6)

These critical incidents make patients' families and even clinicians distressed, which may lead to very serious implications for the corresponding hospitals. If proper measures are not taken, the factors that risk communication in Hong Kong EDs could be inherent in everyday medical practices (Pun et al., 2015).

Handover: Time pressures and high patient loads in ED context

A lot of ED clinicians in Hong Kong face time pressures as well as high patient loads (Pun et al., 2015). Pun et al. (2015) found that the ED they studied involved two or more doctors discussing their patients in brief terms during a clinical handover. During this doctor-doctor conversation, the interviewees said they tended to converse in short and informal sentences verbally, either in Cantonese or code-switch between spoken Cantonese and English. They also shared that they would also write English written notes during this type of handover. They would document in a condensed format repleted with tick boxes that lacked a focus on the details about a patient's changing condition. A doctor found clinical handovers and extensive documentation quite impractical in local EDs because the high demand for emergency services and the consequential time pressures:

> *We have 600 patients a day . . .. So it would be very difficult for us to do a formal handover between doctors and nurses. So we just do some mini-handovers between the doctors themselves, and the nurses will also do some handovers among themselves.* (INT_Doc_7)

The lack of interpersonal interactions

In Pun et al.'s (2015) study, while most of the interviewees recognised the significance of implementing patient-centred care and the relevant principles, the high-stress environment of their workplace inevitably made them feel too busy or not comfortable enough to actively engage in communication. Only a minor number of the interviewees felt capable of showing empathy to their patients or spending time to reassure them of the quality of their care. Therefore, these ED interviewees minimised their patients' participation during consultations and decision-making processes about treatments, in turn deemphasising the significance of expressing empathy through interpersonal communication (Slade et al., 2015a; 2015b). Therefore, interpersonal communication skills and measures taken or training sessions offered by local hospitals that help clinicians in this area require improvement.

How to tackle these issues and build trusting relationships between ED clinicians and patients

While there are existing studies that reported on the nature and frequency of the occurrences of communication issues during conversations with foreign-language-speaking patients (Frank, 2000; Bischoff et al., 2003; Hudelson & Vilpert, 2009) or patients who come from different cultural backgrounds (Vasquez & Javier, 1991; Brooks, 1992; Timmins, 2002; Alegrıa et al., 2009), a limited number of them discussed clinician's responses to communication needs in a rapid and high-stress environment like EDs in multilingual context

(Chandler et al., 2015; Pun et al., 2015; Slade et al., 2016). In order to address such a knowledge gap, Slade et al. (2015a; 2015b) advised communication training programmes for ED staff that are designed to improve the quality of medical communication in order to lower the number of patient complaints, avoid adverse incidents, and higher clinicians' confidence and satisfaction. Slade et al. (2015a) developed a communication framework for ED clinicians to build rapport with and explain medical concepts to their patients in Hong Kong settings. Pun et al. (2015) also explored the discourse strategies that local ED clinicians to show empathy to their patients. The study built on Slade et al.'s research (2015b) to list the strategies used by clinicians to promote the sharing of medical knowledge and effective decision-making processes, which are (1) creating the space for patients to talk about their stories; (2) seeking and acknowledging patients' knowledge of and perspectives towards their medical conditions; (3) explaining medical concepts to patients through shifting between medical and layman language; and (4) talking to patients about their diagnoses and treatments using direct and clear terms. Table 10.1 includes details about the stated strategies.

Effective communication between healthcare providers and patients plays a crucial role in fostering shared medical knowledge and facilitating informed decision-making. The strategies outlined in Table 10.1 provide a structured approach to enhancing patient engagement, ensuring they understand their medical conditions and empowering them to participate actively in their treatment plans.

One of the fundamental strategies is *encouraging patient narratives*, which involves creating an open and welcoming space for patients to share their experiences, symptoms and concerns. When doctors invite patients to describe their health issues in detail, it not only helps in accurate diagnosis but also makes the patient feel heard and valued. For instance, asking an open-ended question such as 'Could you walk me through what's been going on with your sleep lately?' allows the patient to provide a more comprehensive account of their symptoms, leading to a more informed and collaborative discussion.

Another key aspect of patient-centred communication is *acknowledging patient knowledge*. Patients often have insights about their own health based on previous experiences or research, and recognising this knowledge fosters a sense of partnership in care. When a doctor acknowledges a patient's effort, such as discussing dietary changes for digestion issues, it validates the patient's role in managing their health and encourages them to actively participate in treatment decisions.

Table 10.1 Key Communication Strategies for Shared Medical Knowledge and Decision-making (adapted from Slade 2015 with Examples from the local Data)

Communication Strategy	Description	Example of Talk
Encouraging Patient Narratives	Foster an open and comfortable environment where patients feel free to describe their symptoms and health concerns.	**Doctor:** 'Could you walk me through what's been going on with your sleep lately?' **Patient:** 'I've 'been waking up several times at night, and it's making me feel exhausted during the day.'
Acknowledging Patient Knowledge	Validate and incorporate the patient's understanding of their symptoms and previous treatments to encourage active participation in their care.	**Doctor:** 'You mentioned trying a new diet for your digestion issues. How has that been working for you?' **Patient:** 'I think it's helped a little, but I still get bloated in the evenings.'
Normalising Patient Concerns	Reassure patients that their symptoms or reactions are common, reducing unnecessary anxiety.	**Patient:** 'I keep getting these headaches in the afternoon. Is that something to worry about?' **Doctor:** 'That's actually quite common when adjusting to new medication. Let's keep an eye on it and see if it improves.'
Using Clear, Direct Language	Avoid complex medical terminology and provide simple, straightforward explanations for better patient comprehension.	**Doctor:** 'Your blood pressure is a little high today, which means your heart is working harder than it should. We'll discuss ways to lower it.'
Providing Comprehensive Explanations	Offer detailed guidance on the diagnosis, treatment and next steps to ensure clarity and adherence.	**Doctor:** 'I'll give you an inhaler to use when you feel short of breath. Just take one puff, wait a minute, then take another if needed.' **Patient:** 'Should I use it every day?' **Doctor:** 'No, only when you're feeling tightness in your chest or struggling to breathe.'

Normalising patient concerns is essential for alleviating anxiety and reassuring patients that certain symptoms or side effects are common and manageable. When a patient expresses worry about a recurring symptom, such as headaches, a doctor's response that frames the issue as typical – rather than alarming – can ease their concerns while still providing medical guidance. This reassurance helps build trust and ensures that patients remain engaged in their care without unnecessary distress. To further support understanding, healthcare providers should prioritise using clear, direct language. Medical jargon can be intimidating and confusing for patients, making it difficult for them to fully grasp their condition and treatment options. Simple, non-technical explanations – such as clarifying that high blood pressure means the heart is working harder than usual – ensure that patients can follow medical advice and make informed choices regarding their health.

Finally, *providing comprehensive explanations* ensures that patients receive the necessary details about their diagnosis, treatment, and next steps. Clear and structured guidance, like explaining when and how to use an inhaler, eliminates uncertainty and improves adherence to medical recommendations. By offering step-by-step instructions and confirming patient understanding, doctors enhance patient confidence in managing their own health. In summary, these communication strategies are essential in bridging the gap between medical expertise and patient understanding. By fostering open dialogue, acknowledging patient knowledge and ensuring clarity, healthcare providers can enhance patient participation, improve health outcomes and build stronger doctor-patient relationships.

To conclude, taking into account the traditional Chinese values that shape Hong Kong's high-risk clinical environments, ICU and ED clinicians are encouraged to prioritise human factors and patient-centred values rather than solely focusing on conflict management. In the ICU, fostering a culture of communication openness is particularly crucial, as clinicians must feel safe and empowered to speak up in order to ensure patient safety and enhance teamwork within the unit. Additionally, this chapter has highlighted the importance of understanding the broad scope of both medical and non-medical communication in ICU settings, particularly regarding the needs of mechanically ventilated (MV) patients, whose voices often go unheard. By recognising the multidimensional nature of communication – including medical discussions, emotional support and decision-making – ICU clinicians can facilitate more holistic patient care.

Beyond the ICU, this chapter has also examined the significant communication challenges faced by clinicians in another high-risk setting: Emergency Departments (EDs) in Hong Kong. The findings illustrate how linguistic complexity, repeated translations, inconsistencies in medical documentation and hierarchical pressures contribute to communication barriers. Given the trilingual nature of Hong Kong's healthcare system, these challenges necessitate structured strategies to enhance communication effectiveness. The proposed framework for multilingual ED clinicians aims to facilitate patient-centred communication practices, ensuring that shared medical knowledge and decision-making processes are more efficient and equitable.

The discussion of communication challenges in high-risk clinical settings naturally extends to primary care, where doctor-patient interactions are equally complex and culturally influenced. The following chapter shifts focus to the role of doctor-patient communication in primary care within the Chinese cultural context. It explores how language barriers, cultural values and asymmetrical power dynamics impact communication and decision-making in primary care consultations. By examining these challenges and proposing strategies for building trust, managing patient expectations and enhancing cultural competence, Chapter 11 offers insights into improving communication in less acute yet equally critical healthcare settings.

11

The role of doctor-patient communication in primary care within the Chinese cultural context

Effective communication between doctors and patients is a critical component of delivering high-quality healthcare and achieving positive clinical outcomes, particularly in primary care setting. In this setting, long-term relationships, continuity of care, and the management of chronic conditions are essential to patient well-being (Deledda et al., 2013). As primary care is often the first point of contact for patients, communication plays a vital role in building trust, ensuring patient satisfaction, and fostering adherence to treatment plans (Slade et al., 2015a). For an example, a patient visits a primary care doctor with symptoms of high blood pressure. Only through clear communication, the doctor explains the condition, addresses concerns and collaborates on a treatment plan, building trust and ensuring the patient adheres to the prescribed care. For these reasons, communication training has become increasingly recognised as a key element in equipping healthcare professionals with the skills needed to navigate the unique challenges of primary care, especially within culturally diverse populations (Pun et al., 2018).

In primary care, effective doctor-patient communication extends beyond basic information exchange; it is central to delivering patient-centred care (Rider et al., 2014). Research has consistently shown that good doctor-patient communication correlates with improved health outcomes, including patient satisfaction, treatment adherence and better management of chronic conditions (Slade et al., 2015; Stewart, 1995; Pun et al., 2018). However, primary care presents distinct challenges in delivering effective communication. These include managing patient expectations, addressing the complexities of chronic illnesses and overcoming barriers related to cultural and linguistic diversity (Slade et al., 2016). For instance, in Hong Kong, doctors often communicate with patients in Cantonese or Mandarin, while recording the patient's medical conditions in English. Research has highlighted the risks associated with these bilingual exchanges, as potential miscommunications may occur when patient information is transferred across different stages of care and languages (Pun et al., 2015; 2016a; 2016b; Pun, 2021a; 2021b; 2022). What makes the communication at primary care more complicated from other cultural contexts, doctors may face communication challenges due to the traditional Chinese cultural norms and practices (Pun et al., 2018). In the Chinese cultural context, additional factors, such as family involvement in decision-making (i.e. decision-making for cancer patients is often controlled by family over patient's individual preference) and the cultural importance of 'face' in doctor-patient interactions, further complicate the dynamics of communication (Jin, 2019; Pun et al., 2018).

This chapter explores these challenges in the context of primary care in the Chinese context, presenting evidence-based strategies which documented in the literatures for enhancing doctor-patient communication. It will examine techniques for building trust and rapport with patients, approaches for managing expectations in treatment plans and specialised communication skills required for managing chronic diseases. Furthermore, the following section will address the importance of cultural competence, the role of health literacy and the integration of technology in improving patient communication. Through these discussions, healthcare professionals will gain practical insights and strategies to enhance communication, thereby improving patient outcomes in primary care settings, particularly within the Chinese cultural framework.

Challenges to effective communication in primary care

Effective communication in primary care settings is crucial for delivering high-quality healthcare and ensuring positive patient outcomes. However, various factors can impede the process, particularly in high-pressure environments like those in Hong Kong's healthcare system. This section discusses the primary challenges to effective communication, including time constraints, language barriers, cultural factors and asymmetrical power dynamics.

Time constraints

One of the most significant barriers to effective communication in primary care is the limited time available during consultations. Primary care doctors often face immense pressure to manage heavy patient loads, limiting the time they can dedicate to each patient. For instance, in Hong Kong, a primary care doctor seeing sixty patients in a single day might only have five minutes per patient, leaving little time to discuss underlying concerns or explore lifestyle factors that could impact their health, potentially resulting in incomplete care and misunderstandings about treatment plans. This time crunch frequently results in rushed interactions where establishing rapport and thoroughly understanding the patient's concerns becomes difficult (Desmond & Copeland, 2000). Research has shown that time constraints can hinder doctors from fully explaining diagnoses, treatment options or addressing patient concerns in depth, which can result in reduced patient satisfaction and adherence to treatment plans (Fenton et al., 2012; Pun, 2023; Slade et al., 2015a).

The urgency to rapidly collect essential information often results in a directive communication style, where doctors emphasise efficiency at the expense of patient engagement. In these situations, patients may feel that their concerns are being dismissed or inadequately addressed (Pendleton et al., 2003; Vincent & Coulter, 2002). Additionally, the doctor's focus may narrow to immediate symptoms, potentially leading to misdiagnoses if deeper, contextual factors such as lifestyle or psychosocial elements are overlooked. For example, a doctor might quickly ask a patient about their symptoms without allowing time for the patient to share their full medical history or express concerns about their mental well-being. This could result in the doctor misdiagnosing the patient with a straightforward illness, while underlying stress or lifestyle issues remain unaddressed, ultimately impacting the patient's overall health (Maxwell, 2018). To mitigate the impact of time constraints, primary care settings must employ structured communication frameworks, like the Cambridge-Calgary Guide, that allow healthcare professionals to efficiently cover key points without sacrificing the quality of the interaction. The Cambridge-Calgary Guide enhances doctor-patient communication by focusing on a patient-cantered approach, promoting active listening, and ensuring that patients are well-informed and involved in decision-making (Kurtz, 2006; Iversen et al., 2020). It emphasises active listening, patient-centred communication and ensuring patients' understanding of their health issues and treatment plans (Mudiyanse, 2016). It encourages doctors to build rapport with patients, explore their perspectives on their illness and involve them in decision-making (Elwyn et al., 2001). This structure helps to mitigate common barriers in communication, such as misunderstandings and insufficient time to cover key concerns (Kurtz, 2006). This structured method improves the flow of medical consultations, helping doctors to address both the clinical and emotional needs of patients while building trust and understanding. Furthermore, limited time often leaves little room for clarifying any misunderstandings or ensuring that patients fully grasp their diagnosis or treatment plan. This challenge is compounded in multilingual settings, where effective communication requires extra effort to bridge language gaps.

Language barriers

In multilingual societies like Hong Kong, communication in primary care becomes particularly complex. Patients may struggle to articulate their symptoms accurately in a second language, or they may find it challenging to comprehend medical terminology. As Slade et al. (2015) note, Hong Kong's healthcare system often involves multilingual interactions, with frequent code-switching between Cantonese, Mandarin and English. For instance, some patients from mainland China may present medical records written in simplified Chinese, which doctors in Hong Kong may find difficult to interpret, as most medical records in Hong Kong are written in English. Communication challenges can also arise when patients speak only Mandarin, while many doctors primarily communicate in Cantonese or English. These language differences introduce potential risks during translation, especially when conveying information between everyday language and medical terminology in English. This code-switching can lead to misunderstandings, especially when complex medical terms are involved (Pun et al., 2015; Pun, 2022; 2023). Furthermore, patients may misinterpret information due to differences in language proficiency, resulting in confusion and anxiety (Ali & Johnson, 2017).

Conversely, doctors who are not fluent in the patient's preferred language may rely on translators or family members to facilitate communication. While this approach can be helpful, it also carries risks of misinterpretations or omissions of crucial information (Angelelli, 2004; Li et al., 2017). For instance, the patient's description of their symptoms may be inadvertently altered in translation, potentially leading to incorrect diagnoses or treatment plans. This reliance on intermediaries can also affect the level of trust and rapport between doctors and patients, as patients might feel their concerns are not being directly heard by the healthcare provider (Dang et al, 2017). To address language barriers, doctors should consider developing basic proficiency in the languages commonly spoken by their patients or employing trained medical interpreters who understand both the language and cultural context of patients (Carrillo, 1999; Hemberg & Vilander, 2017; Hudelson, 2005; Yeheskel & Rawal, 2019). Additionally, doctors can use simple, non-technical language and visual aids to enhance patients' understanding, thereby reducing the risk of miscommunication.

Cultural factors

Cultural norms play a significant role in shaping doctor-patient communication. In Chinese culture, including those in Hong Kong, there is often an emphasis on deference to authority figures (Pun, 2018). This cultural attitude can affect the dynamics of medical consultations, as patients may be hesitant to express their opinions, ask questions or disagree with the doctor. Instead, they might prioritise family harmony or avoid causing discomfort by withholding information or concerns (Frosch et al., 2012; Pun et al., 2018). Moreover, family involvement in healthcare decisions is a prominent feature in many Chinese culture (Pun et al., 2023). Patients may defer decision-making to family members, creating an additional layer of complexity for doctors seeking to communicate directly with the patient (Hunink et al., 2014). This situation can complicate the exchange of information, as doctors must navigate not only the patient's perspective but also the family's views and expectations.

Medical professionals can develop cultural competence to overcome these barriers, including an understanding of cultural nuances that may affect communication. They should be trained to recognise signs of patient hesitance and employ strategies to create a more open, collaborative environment (Shelley et al., 2009). In the Hong Kong context, some doctors did enhance their cultural competence by understanding the diverse backgrounds of their patients, including the cultural differences between local Cantonese-speaking patients and those from mainland China or different ethnic minority groups or patients from other regions. Training in cultural sensitivity does help doctors recognise subtle signs of patient discomfort or hesitance, such as a reluctance to ask questions or express concerns, particularly in hierarchical or family-centric cultures. By creating a more open, inclusive environment through active listening and patient-cantered communication strategies, medical professionals can foster trust and encourage greater patient engagement (See more from Slade et al., 2015). For example, doctors can invite patients to share their thoughts and concerns, explicitly emphasising that their input is valuable and necessary for effective healthcare. Similarly, acknowledging the role of family in decision-making while gently guiding the patient to express their own preferences can help balance cultural considerations with the need for direct doctor-patient communication.

Asymmetrical power dynamics

The traditional doctor-patient relationship often positions the doctor as the expert and the patient as the passive recipient of information (Beach, 2015; Kaba & Sooriakumaran, 2007). This dynamic can discourage patients from actively participating in their healthcare or voicing their preferences. Research by Slade, Pun, Lock, and Eggins (2016) indicates that this hierarchical structure can result in patients passively accepting medical advice, potentially leaving critical concerns unaddressed. Patients who perceive themselves as having less authority may avoid asking questions, seeking clarification, or challenging the doctor's recommendations, which can negatively affect their adherence to treatment and overall satisfaction (Squier, 1990; Beisecker, 1990; Frosch et al., 2012).

Additionally, this power asymmetry perhaps can create communication risk points where the patient feels sidelined (Pun et al., 2018; Lalonde a& Adler, 2015). For example, if doctors focus primarily on clinical information without engaging the patient in discussions about their personal experiences and perspectives, patients may leave the consultation feeling misunderstood and disempowered. These missed opportunities for dialogue can lead to dissatisfaction and non-compliance with treatment plans (Kemp et al., 1996). To counteract asymmetrical power dynamics, doctors should adopt a shared decision-making model (Charles et al., 1999; Gwyn & Elwyn, 1999). This approach involves inviting patients to participate in their decisions, explaining medical treatment options in accessible language, and validating the patient's concerns and preferences. For example, in a primary care setting in Hong Kong, a doctor treating a patient with hypertension might explain the various treatment options, including lifestyle changes and medication, in simple terms. By asking the patient for their input and discussing the pros and cons of each option, the doctor fosters a collaborative decision-making process that empowers the patient and reduces the sense of hierarchy in the interaction. Using inclusive language, asking open-ended questions, and checking for understanding can help shift the power dynamic towards a more balanced, collaborative interaction (Hsieh et al., 2013). The following section will further explore some communication challenges faced by doctors in primary care context.

Addressing communication challenges in primary care

Recognising the numerous challenges in doctor-patient communication, particularly in the fast-paced and diverse environment of primary care, research has highlighted several strategies to enhance interactions and bridge communication gaps (Aita et al., 2005; Levinson et al., 2010; Rattray et al., 2017; Pun, 2023). These challenges can arise from various factors, including time constraints, language barriers, cultural differences and asymmetrical power dynamics between doctors and patients (Rocque & Leanza, 2015). If doctors communicate without adequate communication strategies, patients may feel misunderstood or disengaged, which can lead to incomplete diagnoses, reduced adherence to treatment plans or compliance to treatments and ultimately poorer health outcomes (Slade et al., 2015). For example, a study on diabetic patients found that when healthcare providers failed to communicate effectively, patients were less likely to adhere to their prescribed treatments or properly manage their condition, leading to poor glycaemic control and increased risks of complications such as cardiovascular disease (Graffigna et al., 2014). Without clear communication, patients may not fully understand their condition or the importance of their treatment plan, resulting in suboptimal health outcomes (Pinelli et al., 2017).

To counter these issues, several communication strategies have been found useful to prioritise mutual understanding, build trust, and foster patient-centred care. These strategies aim to create a more open and empathetic dialogue between doctors and patients, ensuring that the patient's voice is heard and that their concerns, values and preferences are fully considered in the decision-making process (Pun, 2023). By applying these strategies, primary care professionals can enhance the quality of care provided, improve patient satisfaction and help ensure that patients are more engaged and proactive in managing their health. The foundation of these strategies is built on key principles such as active listening, empathy, the use of clear and simple language, shared decision-making and cultural sensitivity (Vranceanu et al., 2009). Together, these strategies can address the diverse needs of patients, from those who face linguistic or cultural challenges, to those managing chronic illnesses, or patients who simply need more time and attention during consultations (Greenhalgh et al., 2006). For example, using clear communication and culturally sensitive approaches can help doctors meet the unique needs of patients with language barriers or chronic conditions, fostering better understanding and engagement in their care.

Implementing these communication strategies is crucial not only for improving individual patient outcomes but also for promoting more effective, patient-cantered healthcare across primary care settings.

Active listening and empathy

One of the foundational aspects of effective communication is active listening paired with empathetic responses (Singh & Dey, 2021). Studies have shown that when patients feel heard and understood, they are more likely to disclose vital information about their symptoms, concerns and personal contexts (Heritage & Maynard, 2006; Slade et al., 2015). For example, a doctor might notice a patient's hesitant tone and slouched posture when discussing their diagnosis, prompting the doctor to acknowledge their concerns by saying, '*It seems like you're feeling uncertain about this; let's talk through any questions you have*'. Active listening involves more than just hearing the patient's words; it includes interpreting non-verbal cues, such as body language and tone of voice, and responding in ways that validate the patient's feelings and experiences (Kee et al., 2018; Lorié et al., 2017).

Doctors can employ several strategies to enhance active listening, including the use of open-ended questions that encourage patients to share their narratives openly (Slade et al., 2015; Pun & Chor, 2020). For example, asking, '*Can you tell me more about how you've been feeling?*' invites patients to elaborate on their symptoms and concerns. Additionally, non-verbal cues like nodding, maintaining eye contact and leaning forward convey attentiveness and interest. Reflecting back on the patient's emotions – for instance, saying, '*It sounds like you're feeling quite worried about this*', – can further demonstrate empathy and build rapport. Such strategies not only help establish trust but also provide doctors with a more comprehensive understanding of the patient's condition, leading to more tailored and effective care plans.

Clear and simple language

One of the most common obstacles to clear communication in primary care setting is the use of medical jargon, which can confuse patients and hinder their understanding of diagnoses and treatment plans. Medical jargon can be a significant barrier to effective communication, particularly in multilingual societies like Hong Kong, where patients may already face challenges in articulating their symptoms in a second language (Slade et al., 2015). To address this, doctors can strive to use clear and simple language when discussing diagnoses, treatment options and medical procedures (Lee et al., 2002).

One possible approach is to break down complex medical concepts into everyday terms and use analogies or visual aids to enhance patient comprehension. For example, when explaining high blood pressure, a Chinese doctor in a primary care setting might compare it to the concept of '*qi*' (vital energy) flowing through the body's meridians, where an excessive buildup of pressure can block the flow, much like how blocked water in a pipe causes strain and potential damage to the system Similarly, using diagrams, charts, or models can provide a visual representation of the condition or treatment, making it easier for patients to grasp. Doctors can also encourage patients to ask questions and provide explanations at a pace that allows for understanding (Lee et al., 2002). Techniques such as the 'teach-back' method, where patients are asked to repeat back the information in their own words, can help ensure that they have accurately understood the key points of their care plan.

Shared decision-making

Shared decision-making is a collaborative process in which doctors involve patients in their medical decisions. This approach not only empowers patients but also enhances their adherence to treatment plans by making them active participants in their care (Hickmann et al., 2022). According to Slade et al. (2015), patients who are engaged in decision-making are more likely to follow through with their treatment, as they feel their values and preferences have been considered. In practice, shared decision-making involves presenting treatment options clearly, discussing potential benefits and risks, and exploring the patient's values, lifestyle and preferences. Doctors can support this process by providing accessible, patient-friendly resources, such as brochures or reputable online information, that patients can review at their own pace (Ho et al., 2024). For example, a doctor treating a patient with type two diabetes might present several treatment options, such as adjusting diet, increasing physical activity or starting medication. The doctor would explain the potential benefits and risks of each option, such as the possible side effects of medication versus the lifestyle changes required for non-pharmaceutical approaches. By discussing the patient's daily routine, cultural dietary preferences and willingness to commit to lifestyle adjustments, the doctor and patient can collaboratively decide on the best treatment plan that aligns with the patient's values and needs. This step is especially important when dealing with chronic conditions, where long-term management requires patient commitment and understanding (Morgan et al., 2017). Additionally, doctors should invite patients to voice their opinions and ask questions, explicitly conveying that their input is valued (Pun, 2023). For example, asking, *'How do you feel about starting this new medication?'* can open a dialogue that not only clarifies the patient's perspective but also reinforces their role in the decision-making process.

Cultural sensitivity

Cultural factors play a pivotal role in shaping patients' perceptions of illness, communication styles and attitudes towards healthcare decisions. In Chinese cultures, including Hong Kong, values such as deference to authority, respect for hierarchy and the emphasis on family harmony significantly influence doctor-patient interactions (Cong, 2004; Slade et al., 2015; Pun et al., 2020; 2021; Xiao et al., 2020). Given these cultural nuances, it is essential for medical professionals to adopt communication strategies that are culturally sensitive, recognising and respecting the beliefs, values, and preferences of patients. A review by Pun et al. (2018) highlights the complexity of clinician-patient communication across East Asia, stressing the need for a culturally tailored health communication model that takes into account local practices, family involvement, and communication preferences. Such a model is vital for fostering trust, improving decision-making, and enhancing patient satisfaction. While research in the region is gradually moving beyond Western-centric communication frameworks, Pun emphasises that more work is needed to fully address the region's unique cultural attitudes towards healthcare and develop approaches that align with the specific needs of Chinese patients.

Cultural sensitivity involves taking the time to understand the patient's cultural background and how it might impact their health beliefs and behaviours (Schouten & Meeuwesen, 2006). For instance, when discussing sensitive topics like death and dying, doctors should be mindful of cultural norms that may discourage open conversation about such matters. By acknowledging and showing respect for these cultural nuances, doctors can facilitate a more open and comfortable dialogue with their patients. For example, a Chinese doctor in a primary care setting might use indirect language such as *focusing on comfort and quality of life* instead of explicitly discussing death, allowing the conversation to align with cultural sensitivities and making the patient and family feel more at ease. In practical terms, doctors may start by asking open-ended questions about the patient's cultural or religious beliefs that might influence their care preferences (Shrank et al., 2005; Pun et al., 2020; 2021). This approach not only shows respect for the patient's background but also provides insight into how the doctor can tailor their communication and recommendations to be more culturally appropriate (Paternotte et al., 2015). Moreover, being aware of non-verbal communication differences across cultures, such as eye contact and gestures, can help doctors navigate interactions more effectively. For example, doctors in Chinese context might avoid prolonged eye contact, recognising that in Chinese culture it can be perceived as disrespectful or confrontational, thereby creating a more comfortable and respectful environment for the patient (Pun, 2023). This reflects the importance of developing robust communication skills that are not only culturally sensitive but also adaptable to a variety of patient needs. To ensure that medical professionals are equipped to handle these nuances, continuous communication skills training is essential.

Communication skills training for cultural differences

Given the complexity of primary care communication, continuous training in communication skills is essential for medical professionals. Research emphasises that such training should encompass techniques for navigating cultural differences, managing time effectively and employing strategies for clear and empathetic communication (Amutio-Kareaga et al., 2017; Larson & Yao, 2005; Slade et al., 2015). Communication skills training programmes can include role-playing scenarios, workshops on cultural competence, and modules on active listening and patient engagement techniques (Holcomb et al., 2022; Rønning & Bjørkly, 2019). For example, training sessions could simulate consultations with patients from different cultural backgrounds, helping doctors practise adapting their communication style to diverse needs. Similarly, courses on managing time during consultations can provide doctors with tools to prioritise discussions, ensuring that even within a limited timeframe, patients feel heard and involved in their care (Zulman et al., 2020; Tongue et al., 2005). For instance, Chinese doctors in primary care might engage in training sessions where they practise communicating with patients who prefer family-centred decision-making, learning how to involve family members while ensuring the patient's voice is still central in time-limited consultations.

Incorporating intercultural communication skills training into medical education and ongoing professional development can help doctors build the necessary competencies to address the various challenges due to cultural differences they encounter in primary care settings (Levinson et al., 2010). By honing these skills, medical professionals can foster stronger doctor-patient relationships, improve patient satisfaction and ultimately enhance health outcomes (Goold & Lipkin, 1999). With effective communication skills as a foundation, doctors can better navigate the complexities of patient interactions in primary care settings. However, building trust and rapport with patients extends beyond mastering individual techniques; it requires a holistic approach to managing patient expectations, addressing chronic conditions and adapting to cultural nuances (Kress et al., 2015; Martini, 2018; Slade et al., 2015). By applying the principles learned through continuous communication training, medical professionals, particularly for primary care doctors, can foster meaningful relationships with their patients. The following section explores how trust-building, cultural competence, health literacy and technology utilisation play vital roles in enhancing communication and patient care in the primary care context.

Building trust and rapport in primary care

Effective communication is fundamental to building trust and fostering a therapeutic relationship between doctors and patients. Trust serves as the foundation upon which patients feel safe to express their concerns, seek advice and adhere to treatment plans (Mechanic & Schlesinger, 1996). In primary care, where patients often seek care for a wide range of chronic and acute conditions, the importance of trust cannot be overstated. Trust allows patients to feel confident in their doctor's expertise and to engage in open dialogue about sensitive or stigmatised health issues, particularly within the Chinese cultural context where patients may hesitate to share personal information or express emotions openly (Mechanic & Meyer, 2000). Moreover, in Chinese culture, trust in medical professionals is often intertwined with respect for authority and social hierarchy (Pun, 2023). Patients may defer to doctors as figures of authority, which can facilitate trust but also pose challenges if communication is too one-sided. Building a relationship that encourages not only respect but also collaboration is critical in overcoming this potential imbalance. This section explores key strategies for enhancing trust and rapport in the primary care setting, such as managing patient expectations, addressing chronic conditions, practising cultural competence, enhancing health literacy and utilising technology for patient engagement. These approaches help to bridge the gap between the doctor's role as an authority figure and the patient's need for personal agency in managing their health.

Developing trusting relationships

The nature of primary care, characterised by regular and ongoing interactions, provides a unique opportunity for doctors to establish strong, trust-based relationships with their patients. Trust develops through consistent use of techniques such as active listening, empathy and providing clear, transparent explanations. When patients feel heard and understood, they are more likely to share their health concerns openly, resulting in more accurate diagnoses and effective treatment plans (Street et al., 2009). For example, a patient initially visits their primary care doctor for headaches, but after feeling heard and understood through the doctor's active listening, they disclose additional symptoms like fatigue and chest tightness. This leads the doctor to diagnose stress-induced hypertension rather than treating the headaches in isolation, resulting in a more accurate diagnosis and effective treatment plan.

Active listening, in particular, plays a crucial role in building rapport. It involves not only hearing patients' words but also responding in ways that validate their experiences and emotions (Weger et al., 2014). By using open-ended questions, summarising what patients have shared, and reflecting on their emotions, doctors demonstrate a genuine concern for their patients' well-being (Slade et al., 2015). For example, a doctor might say, '*It sounds like you're feeling overwhelmed by these symptoms. Let's talk about how we can manage them together.*' Such responses can significantly enhance patients' trust, making them more likely to adhere to treatment recommendations. By fostering trust and rapport through active listening and empathetic communication, primary care doctors can create a foundation for open dialogue, which is essential for managing patient expectations and ensuring that patients have a clear understanding of their treatment plans moving forward.

Managing patient expectations

A key aspect of building trust is managing patients' expectations regarding their care. In primary care settings, doctors can clearly communicate the benefits and limitations of treatments, particularly when dealing with chronic illnesses where a cure may not be possible, and management is ongoing. In the Chinese context, where patients and their families often hold high expectations for successful treatment, especially when consulting with medical professionals seen as authority figures, it becomes even more crucial for doctors to carefully set realistic expectations (Pun, 2023). Research indicates that patients who have a realistic understanding of their condition and the expected outcomes are more likely to be satisfied with their care and comply with treatment plans (Bowling et al., 2013). For example, when discussing a chronic condition like diabetes, a doctor might explain that while the condition cannot be 'cured', it can be effectively managed with lifestyle changes and medication.

Besides, some Chinese doctors might also prefer engaging the family in understanding the treatment plan for chronic illnesses, emphasising the long-term nature of management to help align expectations and support the patient's adherence (Pun, 2023). By setting realistic expectations, doctors help patients prepare for the long-term nature of their condition, which can foster a more proactive approach to self-care. Additionally, being upfront about potential side effects, the frequency of follow-up visits, and the possibility of adjustments to the treatment plan helps patients understand the full scope of their care, reducing the risk of future misunderstandings or dissatisfaction. By effectively managing patient expectations, particularly in the context of chronic illnesses, doctors lay the groundwork for addressing these long-term conditions in a collaborative and patient-centred manner, which is essential for ensuring sustained engagement and successful outcomes in primary care.

Addressing chronic conditions

Managing chronic conditions such as diabetes, hypertension and asthma requires ongoing communication between doctors and patients (Østbye et al., 2005). These interactions are not limited to treatment plans; they encompass patient education, progress monitoring, addressing concerns and modifying care strategies as needed. Effective communication empowers patients to take an active role in managing their health, which can lead to better adherence and improved outcomes (Trummer et al., 2006). For example, a patient with asthma may frequently experience flare-ups, but through ongoing communication, the doctor can assess triggers, adjust the medication dosage, provide education on inhaler use and recommend lifestyle changes, helping the patient gain better control of their condition and reduce future attacks.

Doctors can employ a patient-centred approach when addressing chronic conditions, focusing on collaborative goal-setting and problem-solving (Slade et al., 2015). For instance, during follow-up visits, doctors can involve patients in reviewing their progress and adjusting their treatment plan as necessary. Statements like, '*How do you feel about increasing your physical activity as part of managing your blood pressure*?' invite patients to participate in their care decisions, making them feel more invested in the process. Besides, educating patients about self-management is another critical component (Burckhardt, 2005). This includes explaining how lifestyle choices, such as diet and exercise, impact their condition and teaching them how to monitor symptoms effectively. Providing patients with accessible resources, such as written materials or online tools, can further support their understanding and engagement in their care. This empowerment can result in patients taking greater ownership of their health, leading to increased adherence to treatment plans and, ultimately, better health outcomes. By fostering patient engagement and empowering individuals to take an active role in managing chronic conditions, doctors can enhance treatment adherence and improve health outcomes, creating a strong foundation for addressing the cultural factors that further influence patient care in diverse settings such as Hong Kong.

Mastering cultural competence in primary care

Cultural factors significantly influence health beliefs, communication styles and decision-making processes, especially in diverse societies like Hong Kong. Understanding these factors is essential for building rapport, avoiding misunderstandings and providing culturally sensitive care (Carrillo, 1999). In some Chinese families, for example, there may be an expectation for family members' involvements in medical consultations, and patients may defer decision-making to family members as part of maintaining harmony (Slade et al., 2015; Pun et al., 2018). Besides, doctors should be aware of how cultural differences impact patient expectations and communication preferences (Schouten & Meeuwesen, 2006). In fact, cultural competence, in many cultural contexts, involves actively learning about and respecting patients' cultural backgrounds, beliefs and values (Henderson et al., 2018). For instance, in Chinese context, a patient might consult their family members before consenting to a medical procedure or treatment, so doctors should ensure they give time and space for family discussions to support the patient's decision-making process.

When discussing sensitive topics, such as end-of-life care, doctors, particularly, those in the primary care, serving as patient's family doctor, can approach these conversations with cultural sensitivity (Pun et al., 2020; 2021). For instance, understanding that some patients may prefer indirect communication about terminal diagnoses can help doctors navigate these discussions more respectfully (Evans et al., 2006). To practise cultural competence, primary care doctors can ask open-ended questions about patients' beliefs and preferences. Questions like

'*How does your family usually make decisions about health matters?*' or '*How do your cultural beliefs influence your views on treatment options?*' provide valuable insights into the patient's cultural context and can guide the doctor in delivering care that aligns with the patient's values. This approach not only helps avoid potential conflicts but also strengthens the doctor-patient relationship by showing respect for the patient's cultural perspective, particularly for Chinese context. By embracing cultural competence, doctors can build stronger relationships with their patients and deliver care that respects cultural values, paving the way for the next critical aspect of effective communication in primary care: ensuring patients have the health literacy necessary to understand and manage their health conditions (Koehn & Swick, 2006).

Understanding your patient's health literacy levels in order to tailor communication effectively

Health literacy is a vital element of patient empowerment and effective communication. For patients to actively participate in their care, they must have a clear understanding of their health conditions, treatment plans and medications (Schulz & Nakamoto, 2013). However, literacy levels vary widely, particularly true in Chinese context, and many patients find it difficult to navigate complex medical terminology or instructions. As a result, many Chinese patients tend to follow doctors' instructions without question, as they struggle to navigate the complexities of medical information (Pun, 2023). In the Chinese context, where traditional beliefs and practices such as the use of traditional Chinese medicine such as herbal medicine may coexist with modern treatments in primary context, doctors need to clearly explain how conventional medications interact with traditional remedies to prevent misunderstandings and ensure adherence to treatment plans (Pun & Wong, 2022). To overcome these challenges, doctors can prioritise the use of clear, jargon-free language and reinforce verbal explanations with visual aids such as diagrams, charts or models (Slade et al., 2015). One effective strategy is the 'teach-back' method, where patients are asked to restate the information in their own words to ensure comprehension (Shersher et al., 2021). For example, after explaining a new medication regimen, a primary care doctor might say, '*To make sure everything is clear, can you explain how you'll take this medication each day*?' Customising communication to suit each patient's level of understanding is essential for supporting informed patient's participatory decision-making (Epstein et al., 2004). When patients fully grasp their health status and treatment options, they are more likely to adhere to their care plans and engage in behaviours that promote better health outcomes (Street Jr et al., 2009). Transitioning from the importance of health literacy, which focuses on clear communication and patient understanding, technology offers additional solutions to address these challenges by facilitating continuous engagement and support for patients.

Utilising technology for better patient engagement

The integration of technology in healthcare has opened new avenues for enhancing communication and patient education in primary care. Telemedicine and electronic health records (EHRs) are powerful tools that can support ongoing patient engagement and improve access to care (Pawelek et al., 2022). In Hong Kong, the adoption of telemedicine has been gradually expanding, particularly after the Covid-19 pandemic, while EHR systems such as the Electronic Health Record Sharing System (eHRSS) are being increasingly utilised to streamline information sharing and enhance patient management between public and private care (Ong, 2023).

Telemedicine enables remote consultations, making healthcare more accessible for patients who may have difficulty attending in-person visits due to geographical, physical or time constraints (Kvedar et al., 2014). It provides a platform for follow-up consultations, medication reviews and health education, fostering continuity of care (Arsenault et al., 2024). For instance, through telemedicine, doctors can monitor patients' progress and address concerns without requiring them to travel, which can be especially beneficial for those managing chronic conditions. In Hong Kong, primary care doctors have increasingly used telemedicine to follow up with elderly patients, particularly those in remote areas or nursing homes, providing virtual consultations to assess their health status, adjust medications and coordinate care without the need for in-person visits (Yin Choi et al., 2021; Pun 2023). Besides, electronic health records facilitate information sharing between medical professionals and patients. They provide a centralised platform where patients can access their medical history, lab results and treatment plans, promoting transparency and self-management (Simon et al., 2009). EHRs can also be used to send reminders for appointments or medication refills, helping patients stay on track with their care (Car et al., 2017). In Hong Kong, primary care doctors have utilised electronic health records to engage patients by sharing test results, treatment plans and personalised health advice, encouraging patients to take a more active role in managing their health (Wong & Cheung, 2019). By utilising these technological tools, doctors can enhance patient education and engagement, making patients more proactive partners in managing their health.

*

To conclude, effective communication in primary care is a multifaceted challenge, shaped by various factors ranging from time constraints to cultural considerations. The insights presented in this chapter highlight the complexities inherent in doctor-patient interactions and the need for adaptable communication strategies to meet the diverse needs of patients in primary care settings. The identified communication challenges, such as limited consultation time, language barriers, cultural factors, and asymmetrical power dynamics, illustrate the intricate nature of primary care. Each of these challenges can significantly impact patient outcomes, satisfaction, and adherence to treatment plans. Similarly, language barriers can hinder patients' understanding of medical information, particularly in multilingual societies like Hong Kong, where doctors and patients may have varying levels of proficiency in different languages. In Chinese context, cultural factors further complicate interactions, as patients' beliefs, values and expectations around healthcare often differ, requiring doctors to adopt culturally sensitive communication practices.

Despite these challenges, the strategies discussed in this chapter provide a roadmap for primary care professionals to enhance their communication skills and foster stronger doctor-patient relationships. Techniques such as active listening and empathy are foundational to building trust and rapport. When patients feel heard and validated, they are more likely to openly share their concerns and adhere to treatment plans. This is particularly crucial in managing chronic conditions, where patient engagement in long-term self-management is a key determinant of successful outcomes. Furthermore, the chapter emphasises the importance of clear, simple language in medical consultations. Simplifying complex medical concepts, using visual aids and employing the teach-back method can significantly improve patients' understanding of their conditions and treatments. This is especially important in primary care, where patients often encounter a range of health issues and may have varying levels of health literacy. The need for shared decision-making is also a central theme. Patients who are involved in their healthcare decisions tend to have higher satisfaction and adherence rates, as they feel empowered and respected in their care. By presenting treatment options, discussing potential risks and benefits and exploring patient preferences, doctors can cultivate a more collaborative dynamic that shifts the traditional power imbalance in doctor-patient relationships.

This chapter also underscores the critical role of cultural competence in primary care communication. Recognising and respecting cultural differences, including the influence of family in healthcare decisions, is vital for effective communication. Addressing cultural factors is not just about avoiding misunderstandings; it is about providing care that aligns with patients' values and beliefs, thereby improving the overall patient experience. Given the evolving nature of healthcare and the diversity of patients' needs, ongoing training in active listening, cultural competence, time management and patient engagement is crucial. As primary care continues to evolve with technological advancements and increasingly diverse patient populations, the need for adaptable, empathetic communication becomes ever more critical in delivering high-quality healthcare. Effective communication is not a static skill but an ongoing process that requires flexibility, cultural awareness and a commitment to patient engagement.

While this chapter has explored doctor-patient communication in primary care, the principles of effective interaction and structured communication are equally vital in hospital settings, particularly during nursing handovers. The next chapter shifts focus to the role of communication in clinical handovers among nurses in the Chinese context, examining how hierarchical structures, cultural norms and time constraints shape information exchange and impact patient safety. By exploring these dynamics, the next chapter will provide insights into strategies for improving handover communication and ensuring continuity of care.

12

The role of communication at clinical handovers among nurses in the Chinese context

Nursing handover is one of the most critical communicative events in hospital, where responsibility and accountability for patient care are transferred from one nurse to another at the end of each shift (Anderson et al., 2015; Bruton et al., 2016). This moment marks the intersection of patient care continuity, risk management, and team collaboration. The quality of communication during this transfer is essential, as it can significantly impact patient's clinical outcomes, including the prevention of medical errors, the timely administration of treatments and the seamless transition of care plans (Pun et al., 2020a). Poor communication at clinical handovers has been identified as a major contributing factor to avoidable incidents and adverse outcomes in healthcare settings globally (Eggins et al., 2016). Therefore, ensuring clear, structured and comprehensive communication during handover is paramount to patient safety and quality care.

In Chinese contexts, particularly in Mainland China and Hong Kong, the practice of nursing handover is shaped by a unique interplay of hierarchical organisational structures, cultural norms and the complex, fast-paced nature of hospital environments (Pun, 2023a). These factors influence not only the content of the handovers but also the manner in which communication occurs between healthcare professionals (Pun, 2021a). For example, the hierarchical nature of hospital systems together with Chinese culture in Hong Kong often results in junior nurses being reluctant to ask questions or clarify uncertainties during handover, potentially leading to gaps in critical information transmission (Pun, 2023c). Similarly, cultural values emphasising respect for authority and the avoidance of conflict can further inhibit open dialogue at handovers, making it challenging for nurses to engage in communication interactively which is necessary for effective handovers (Eggins & Slade, 2015).

Moreover, the hospital environment in Hong Kong is increasingly dynamic, with high patient loads, short staff-patient interaction times and the growing demands of an ageing population (Pun, 2021b). These conditions add layers of complexity to the already intricate process of handover communication, requiring nurses to be highly proficient in both clinical knowledge and communication skills (Burgess et al., 2020). As healthcare systems in Chinese contexts continue to evolve and modernise, the importance of refining handover practices becomes even more pressing. Research shows that structured communication protocols, such as the ISBAR (Introduction, Situation, Background, Assessment and Recommendation) framework, have been instrumental in improving handover quality by providing a standardised format for information exchange (Eggins et al., 2016; Pun, 2021a). However, while ISBAR offer a valuable tool to nurses for ensuring the quality of communication at handovers, it does not fully address the cultural and interpersonal dynamics that shape handover communication in Chinese healthcare settings (Pun et al., 2018).

This chapter explores the multifaceted role of communication in nursing handover within the Chinese context, examining the ways in which cultural norms, organisational hierarchy and interpersonal dynamics shape the effectiveness of information transfer. It emphasises how these factors can either facilitate or hinder the clear exchange of patient clinical information, which is crucial for ensuring patient safety and continuity of care. Additionally, we identify essential considerations for nurses in the teaching and learning of handover skills, particularly in the environments characterised by rigid hierarchical structures and intense time pressures. By understanding and addressing these cultural and systemic challenges, nursing professionals can adopt best practices that not only enhance communication during handovers but also improve the overall quality of patient care. Furthermore, this chapter outlines strategies for integrating structured communication tools, such as ISBAR, and promoting interactive, patient-centred handovers that empower nurses at all levels to participate actively in the exchange of vital information.

Cultural contexts and communication challenges in nursing handover

In Chinese healthcare systems, entrenched hierarchical structures significantly affect communication during nursing handovers, often limiting the exchange of crucial clinical information. Junior nurses, navigating a complex web of authority, may feel compelled to defer to senior staff, suppressing their ability to engage in open and interactive dialogue – a critical factor for patient safety (Pun,

2023a). Cultural norms prioritising deference to authority and social harmony exacerbate this challenge. As a result, nurses may hesitate to ask questions or seek clarification during handovers, even when important information is unclear. This reluctance to speak up, driven by fear of appearing disrespectful or challenging authority, can lead to incomplete or vague communication, increasing the risk of misunderstandings and errors in patient care (Pun et al., 2021a; 2021b).

In addition to these cultural influences, the organisational environment in Chinese hospitals presents additional challenges for effective handover communication. High patient loads, time pressures and a fast-paced clinical setting leave little room for thorough, interactive communication. Handovers often become rushed processes, where nurses are expected to relay large amounts of critical information within limited time frames (Pun, 2021a). This exacerbates the potential for communication breakdowns, as there may be insufficient time for the receiving nurse to fully comprehend the patient's condition or take necessary follow-up actions.

Several studies have highlighted the unique communication challenges faced by nurses in Hong Kong, where the healthcare system mirrors many of the cultural and hierarchical traits seen in Mainland China (Pun, 2021a; 2021b; 2023a; 2023b; Pun et al., 2018). Research suggests that nursing handovers in Hong Kong are often characterised by a narrative or anecdotal style of communication, where information is conveyed in a descriptive, unstructured manner (Chung et al., 2022; Pun, 2021b). While this storytelling approach may feel natural for some nurses, it introduces significant variability across different staff in the same ward in the way patient information is presented (Pun, 2023b). The lack of a standardised format means that key details about the patient's latest clinical condition, treatment plan or upcoming care needs may be omitted or inconsistently reported. This variability in communication can lead to critical gaps in the handover process, which in turn heightens the likelihood of errors or omissions in patient care (Pun, 2021a). Moreover, the cultural expectation to maintain 'face' (面子 '*mianzi*') and uphold social harmony often discourages nurses from challenging or questioning their peers or superiors during handovers (Pun, 2021a). This further complicates the process, as vital details may go unclarified, leading to a compromised understanding of the patient's needs (Eggins et al., 2016). The combination of these cultural and organisational factors underscores the need for tailored nursing handover communication training that addresses the specific barriers faced by nurses in these environments. Training programmes should focus on equipping nurses with the confidence and skills to navigate these cultural and organisational barriers (Pun, 2023c). By fostering an environment where speak-up culture is encouraged, regardless of hierarchical position, and by promoting the use of structured communication protocols, healthcare systems in China and Hong Kong can significantly improve the clarity, completeness and safety of nursing handovers (Ng et al., 2017b). Ultimately, addressing these cultural and communication challenges is essential for enhancing the overall quality of patient care and reducing the risk of errors during care transitions.

Communication protocol for structured nursing handover

In a fast-paced and often complex environment such as the hospital, effective communication during nursing handover is essential for ensuring continuity of care and minimising the risk of medical errors. One of the most widely adopted communication tools for structuring communication is the ISBAR protocol (Introduction, Situation, Background, Assessment, Recommendation). This framework has gained significant traction because it provides a standardised approach to organising and delivering patient information in a clear, concise and logical manner (Burgess et al., 2020; Shahid & Thomas, 2018). It helps nurses organise and convey patient information in a clear, logical and systematic way, reducing the potential for miscommunication (Eggins & Slade, 2015). By offering a structured format, ISBAR helps nurses to avoid the common pitfalls of fragmented or incomplete communication that can occur during transitions of care. Using ISBAR has been found effective in a bilingual environment where nurses are expected to communicate more in one language (i.e. English) in addition to their mother tongue (Pun, 2021a; 2021b; 2021c; 2021d; 2023c).

In the 'Introduction' phase, the outgoing nurse identifies themselves and the patient, setting the stage for a focused handover. The 'Situation' element allows the nurse to succinctly describe the patient's current condition, including any immediate concerns. The 'Background' section offers a brief summary of the patient's medical history and relevant contextual information, ensuring that the incoming nurse is aware of any ongoing or chronic issues. The 'Assessment' phase involves the nurse's clinical evaluation of the patient, including vital signs, lab results, follow-up plans and any new developments. Finally, the 'Recommendation' stage allows the outgoing nurse to provide specific guidance on the next steps in care. Both outgoing and incoming nurses are encouraged to clarify during the 'Recommendation' stage so both parties can engage in an interactive dialogue, ensuring that any ambiguities are addressed before ending the handover. Additionally, ISBAR helps mitigate the influence of hierarchical dynamics that are common in Chinese healthcare settings. In these environments, junior nurses may be reluctant to challenge or question senior colleagues, which can lead to unaddressed uncertainties during handovers. By incorporating a Question and Answer section into the 'Recommendation' stage, ISBAR encourages a more open and interactive exchange of information, empowering all nurses, regardless of rank, to seek clarification and confirm their understanding of the patient's status (Eggins & Slade, 2012). This fosters a more collaborative approach to patient care, where communication is not just a one-way transfer of information but a two-way dialogue that promotes shared responsibility and accountability (Shahid & Thomas, 2018).

However, implementing ISBAR effectively requires more than simply introducing a framework. For the protocol to be truly effective, it must be integrated into daily practice in a way that empowers nurses to take an active role in the communication process. This includes fostering an environment where asking questions and clarifying uncertainties is not only encouraged but also expected (Eggins & Slade, 2015; Eggins et al., 2016). Nurses can be trained to engage actively in the handover process, ask clarifying questions, and ensure that the information they are receiving or conveying is both accurate and comprehensive (Pun, 2021a). In contexts such as Hong Kong, where hierarchical relationship and cultural norms may inhibit open dialogue, additional training and support are essential to ensure that all nurses, regardless of seniority, feel confident in using ISBAR to facilitate thorough and accurate information exchange (Pun, 2023a; 2023b; 2023c; 2023d).

The implementation of ISBAR has demonstrated tangible improvements in patient safety and care quality in Hong Kong. Research indicates that the use of structured communication tools like ISBAR leads to a reduction in communication-related errors, which are a leading cause of adverse events in healthcare settings (Eggins et al., 2016). Studies have shown that hospitals and healthcare facilities that adopt the ISBAR framework experience fewer incidents of miscommunication during handovers, as the protocol helps to standardise the way in which patient information is transferred between shifts (Pun, 2023b; Slade et al., 2018 , 2019). Moreover, nurses who can present a clear structure of ISBAR results have better communication flow where important details are not overlooked. This directly impacts on patient outcomes by facilitating timely interventions and appropriate follow-up care (Chien et al., 2022).

Moreover, ISBAR can be made adaptable to various clinical contexts, whether in intensive care units, emergency departments or general wards (Burgess et al., 2020). Its structured nature ensures that it can be applied consistently across different departments and specialties, making it a valuable tool for standardising communication practices throughout an entire healthcare facility (Eggins et al., 2016). This universality is particularly beneficial in large hospital systems where staff members may rotate between different units, as it provides a common language for handover communication, reducing variability and enhancing the overall quality of care. In conclusion, the adoption of communication protocols like ISBAR represents a significant step forward in improving the safety, clarity and efficiency of nursing handovers in China and Hong Kong. By providing a structured framework for the exchange of patient information, ISBAR reduces the risk of errors, promotes transparency and fosters a culture of open communication.

Key communication skills in nursing handover

While structured protocols like ISBAR provide a much-needed framework for organising patient information during handovers, the success of these protocols relies heavily on the interpersonal communication skills of the nurses involved. A standardised format can ensure that the necessary clinical details are conveyed, but it is the quality of the interaction between the outgoing and incoming nurses that ultimately determines the effectiveness of the handover. Effective nursing handovers are more than the mechanical transfer of data – they require a two-way dialogue where both parties are fully engaged in the exchange, clarifying any uncertainties and confirming mutual understanding. This interactive approach is critical in minimising the risk of errors and ensuring seamless continuity of care between shifts. To achieve this, nurses can develop and refine five key communication skills (see more from Eggins et al., 2016), which are illustrated in the following sections: (1) asking questions and clarifying clinical information; (2) providing updated and accurate information; (3) engaging in interactive communication; (4) having active listening and non-verbal cues; and (5) building confidence in communication.

Ask questions and clarify clinical information

One of the most essential skills in a successful handover is the ability to ask questions and clarify any ambiguous or unclear details. Studies have shown that nurses who actively seek clarification during handovers are more likely to have a comprehensive understanding of the patient's condition and care plan, which in turn helps to prevent potential errors in treatment or care (Pun, 2018). However, in hierarchical healthcare systems like those found in Hong Kong, junior nurses often feel inhibited from questioning their senior colleagues due to cultural norms of deference and respect for authority (Pun, 2021b). This reluctance to speak up can result in gaps in communication that compromise patient safety. Therefore, training programmes should prioritise creating an open and supportive environment where all nurses, regardless of seniority, feel empowered to ask questions and seek clarification. Encouraging a culture of open dialogue during handovers is critical to ensuring that important information is fully understood and retained by the receiving nurse.

Provide updated and accurate information

The accuracy and timeliness of the information being shared during handover are equally critical (Eggins & Slade, 2015). Incomplete or outdated information can lead to serious errors, particularly when a patient's condition has changed since the last assessment. Nurses need to ensure that the information they convey is current and reflects the patient's present status, including any recent changes in their condition, ongoing treatment or new concerns. This requires nurses to be diligent in verifying all relevant details before the handover begins. Training should emphasise the importance of cross-checking information, particularly in dynamic hospital environments where patients' conditions can fluctuate rapidly. By teaching nurses to prioritise accuracy and timeliness in their communication, healthcare institutions can significantly reduce the risk of miscommunication and improve the overall quality of patient care (Pun, 2021b).

Engage in interactive communication

A handover should not be a passive, one-way transfer of information from one nurse to another. Instead, it should be an active, two-way conversation where both the outgoing and incoming nurses engage in a meaningful exchange of information (Eggins & Slade, 2015). This interaction is crucial to ensuring that both parties have a clear and thorough understanding of the patient's condition and the care plan moving forward. Providing opportunities for the receiving nurse to ask questions, clarify details and confirm their understanding is essential for preventing misunderstandings and ensuring that no important information is overlooked (Slade et al., 2018, 2019). Furthermore, the outgoing nurse should be open to feedback and questions, fostering an environment of collaboration and shared responsibility for the patient's care (Pun, 2021a). This interactive process strengthens the nurse-to-nurse communication bond and ensures continuity of care that is seamless and aligned with the patient's needs.

Engage in active listening and use non-verbal cues

Beyond asking questions and exchanging verbal information, nurses should also be adept at active listening. Active listening involves fully concentrating on what is being communicated, without distraction, and responding thoughtfully. Nurses can be trained to pick up on both the explicit content of the message and the non-verbal cues that may indicate confusion, hesitation or concerns from the other party. This is particularly important in high-stress clinical environments like Emergency Departments (EDs) or Intensive Care Units (ICUs) where non-verbal communication, such as eye contact, body language and tone of voice, can convey additional layers of meaning (Ng et al., 2017a; Pun, 2023a; 2023b). By mastering active listening and being attuned to non-verbal signals, nurses can more effectively identify areas where additional clarification is needed and ensure that all critical information is fully understood by both parties.

Build confidence in communication

Confidence plays a significant role in effective communication during handovers. Nurses who are confident in their communication abilities are more likely to engage in meaningful dialogue, ask the necessary questions and provide thorough explanations. In contrast, those who feel uncertain or intimidated by the power asymmetries in healthcare may refrain from fully participating in the handover process. To address this, training programmes should focus on building communication confidence among nurses (Pun, 2023c). This can be achieved through role-playing exercises, simulations and mentorship opportunities where nurses practise delivering handovers in a supportive setting. Besides, educators can use a blended learning approach to enhance nursing students' communication skills at clinical handovers which has proved effectively (Chung et al., 2022). Over time, this practice can help nurses feel more self-assured and capable of contributing to a high-quality handover process.

While structured protocols like ISBAR are invaluable for standardising the content of nursing handovers, it is the interpersonal communication skills of the nurses that ultimately determine the success of the interaction (Slade et al, 2018, 2019). By fostering a culture of open dialogue, encouraging clarifying questions, ensuring the provision of accurate and timely information, and promoting active engagement and listening, healthcare systems can significantly enhance the quality of their handovers. Training that emphasises these key communication skills is essential for reducing errors, improving patient outcomes and ensuring the continuity of care.

Key information for clinicians to consider when teaching nursing handover in Chinese context

When developing effective nursing handover training programmes in the Chinese clinical contexts, nurses can account for both the unique cultural dynamics at play and the critical importance of clear, accurate communication. The training should go beyond the procedural aspects of handover, addressing the cultural, interpersonal and organisational challenges that impact communication quality. The following are five key areas of focus for clinicians when teaching nursing handover practices (see more from Eggins et al., 2016; Pun et al., 2018; Pun, 2023a). They are: (1) understanding cultural influences on communication; (2) using structured communication tools such as ISBAR; (3) developing interpersonal communication skills; (4) addressing time pressures and workloads; and (5) building confidence to navigate hierarchies and develop a speak-up culture.

Understanding cultural influences on communication

One of the most significant factors influencing communication during handover in China is the deeply embedded hierarchical structure of the healthcare system. Cultural norms that emphasise deference to seniority and respect for authority can inhibit junior nurses from asking questions or challenging information provided by more experienced staff, even when they suspect errors or need clarification. These dynamics, driven by traditional Confucian values of hierarchy and harmony, can lead to communication gaps that compromise patient care (Pun et al., 2018). Therefore, clinicians can educate nurses on how these cultural influences shape communication behaviours. Teaching strategies should focus on creating an environment where open communication is encouraged and normalised, regardless of rank. Nurses should be explicitly trained to ask questions and seek clarification when needed, reframing these actions as essential to patient safety rather than as confrontational or disrespectful. Simulation-based training that mimics real-life power dynamics at workplace can help nurses practise these skills in a controlled setting, empowering them to communicate more effectively in actual handovers (Pun, 2021a; 2021b). This cultural sensitivity in training will help mitigate the risks associated with passive communication, particularly in high-stakes environments.

Using structured communication tools such as ISBAR

To overcome the inherent risks of communication breakdowns, structured communication tools such as ISBAR have proven to be invaluable. By standardising the format of handovers, these tools ensure that all critical patient information is conveyed in a systematic and coherent manner. Clinicians should emphasise the importance of adhering to such protocols during handovers, teaching nurses how to organise and present patient information logically. Training programmes should focus on how to use ISBAR effectively, guiding nurses through each step – starting with a clear introduction, followed by a concise description of the patient's situation, relevant background, clinical assessments and recommended actions. Nurses can also be taught the importance of the 'Question and Answer' component, which encourages interactive dialogue and ensures that any uncertainties are addressed before the handover concludes. This structured approach not only minimises the risk of omissions but also enhances the clarity and precision of the information being communicated (Slade et al., 2018). Structured communication tools provide a reliable framework for organising patient data, particularly in high-pressure situations where time is limited and the risk of errors is heightened.

Developing interpersonal communication skills

While structured communication tools like ISBAR are indispensable, the quality of handovers ultimately hinges on the interpersonal communication skills of the nurses involved. Therefore, clinicians should focus on developing these interpersonal skills in their training programmes. Role-playing exercises and simulations can be particularly effective in this regard, allowing nurses to practise active listening, clarifying questions, and providing feedback in a safe, controlled environment. These exercises can also help nurses become more comfortable with navigating complex conversations, such as those involving difficult or uncertain clinical situations. Research indicates that such training significantly improves the quality of handovers, as it encourages nurses to engage more actively in the process, facilitating clearer and more thorough exchanges of information (Eggins & Slade, 2015; Slade et al., 2018). Additionally, interpersonal communication skills help build trust and rapport between nursing staff, creating a collaborative environment where the quality of patient care is prioritised.

Addressing time pressures and workloads

One of the most pervasive challenges in nursing handovers, particularly in fast-paced hospital environments, is the pressure to complete the handover quickly due to high patient loads and time constraints. Nurses often find themselves juggling multiple patients, leaving little time for comprehensive and detailed handovers. As a result, information may be rushed, incomplete or not communicated at all. Clinicians should teach nurses how to conduct efficient yet thorough handovers, where critical information is prioritised and communicated clearly within a limited timeframe. Training should include strategies for identifying and focusing on the most important patient details, such as changes in condition, key treatment plans and urgent concerns that need immediate attention in the next shift. Nurses should also learn how to manage time effectively during handovers, ensuring that they are not sacrificing the quality of communication due to external pressures (Slade et al., 2018, 2019). By incorporating time management techniques into the training, clinicians can help nurses balance the demands of a high-pressure environment with the need for comprehensive and accurate handovers.

Building confidence to navigate hierarchies and develop a speak-up culture

Lastly, a key aspect of nursing handover training in the Chinese context is fostering the confidence to navigate traditional cultural values and power dynamics within healthcare teams. Nurses, particularly those at the junior level, may feel reluctant to voice concerns or ask questions due to the power dynamics present in many Chinese hospitals. Clinicians should emphasise the importance of assertiveness and confidence in handover situations, teaching nurses that their input is valuable and that seeking clarification is crucial for patient safety. Speak-up culture should be encouraged and fostered when training nursing handover communication (Ng et al., 2017a). Role-playing scenarios that simulate hierarchical interactions can help nurses build the confidence needed to engage more actively during handovers, regardless of the seniority of the other party (Pun, 2023b). By empowering nurses to assert themselves in these settings, clinicians can improve the overall quality of communication and ensure that critical information is shared openly and accurately.

As nursing handovers continue to evolve, the need for efficiency, accuracy and clarity remains paramount. While traditional methods have proven effective, the increasing complexity of healthcare systems and patient needs demands more innovative approaches. Clinicians and healthcare administrators are continually seeking ways to overcome the limitations posed by cultural, linguistic and organisational challenges. In response, advancements in technology, strategies to address language barriers and the inclusion of patients and families in the handover process have emerged as key areas of focus. These developments aim to streamline communication, reduce errors and ensure that the handover process is as seamless and comprehensive as possible. The following sections will explore how these solutions are shaping the future of nursing handover practices.

Technological integration in nursing handover communication

The increasing reliance on digital tools in healthcare has transformed the landscape of communication during nursing handovers. Traditionally, handovers were conducted verbally or with written notes, but the advent of electronic health records (EHRs), telecommunication tools and specialised handover software has streamlined the process, enhancing both the quality and efficiency of information transfer (Troyer & Brady, 2020). Digital technologies enable real-time access to up-to-date patient information, reducing the chances of miscommunication that can occur when data is outdated or inaccurate. EHRs, for example, allow nurses to access comprehensive patient histories, medication records and treatment plans, ensuring that no critical information is omitted during handovers (Forde-Johnston et al., 2023). Telecommunication tools such as secure messaging systems and video conferencing facilitate remote handovers, particularly in large healthcare facilities where direct, face-to-face communication may be challenging.

The benefits of technological integration in nursing handovers are significant. First, it minimises the risk of human error by providing structured templates and automated reminders that ensure all essential aspects of patient care are covered. Second, digital systems often include audit trails, which allow healthcare teams to track and review the information shared during handovers, promoting accountability and transparency. However, there are also challenges to consider. Technical issues, such as system failures or connectivity problems, can disrupt the handover process, potentially leading to delays in patient care. Moreover, data security concerns arise as sensitive patient information is stored and transmitted electronically, making healthcare systems vulnerable to cyberattacks. Nurses can be trained to navigate these systems effectively while adhering to privacy regulations. Another key challenge is the learning curve associated with adopting new technologies. Many nurses, particularly those accustomed to traditional handover methods, may struggle to adapt to digital systems. Ongoing training and support are essential to ensure that all staff members are proficient in using these tools and that the transition to digital handover processes is smooth. While technology offers immense potential for improving the quality and efficiency of nursing handovers, healthcare institutions must address the technical, security and training challenges to fully realise these benefits.

The impact of language proficiency on nursing handover

In bilingual and multilingual contexts like Hong Kong, language proficiency can significantly affect the clarity and effectiveness of communication during nursing handovers. Many nurses in these regions are required to work in both Cantonese and English, the latter being the language of many medical records, international guidelines and communication with non-local staff. Language barriers can lead to misunderstandings, misinterpretation of patient information and omissions during handovers (Pun, 2021b; 2023a). Nurses who are less proficient in the language of communication may struggle to articulate important details, leading to gaps in the transfer of critical information about patient care. Additionally, they may hesitate to ask clarifying questions, fearing embarrassment or misunderstanding, further compounding the risk of errors.

The use of standardised communication tools like ISBAR can help mitigate some of these challenges by providing a structured framework for information exchange. However, without adequate language proficiency, even the most structured protocols can fall short of ensuring effective communication. To address these issues, healthcare institutions must invest in language training programmes for nurses, particularly those working in bilingual environments

(Pun, 2023c). Providing opportunities for nurses to improve their language skills not only enhances the quality of handovers but also boosts their confidence in communicating with colleagues and patients. Additionally, AI-assisted tools and bilingual resources can support nurses during handovers, ensuring that they can accurately convey patient information, regardless of their language proficiency.

Patient involvement in nursing handovers

In recent years, there has been a growing trend towards involving patients and their families in nursing handovers, reflecting the shift towards patient-centred care. Involving patients in handovers such as bed-side nursing handover allows them to participate in discussions about their care, ask questions and clarify any concerns they may have (Eggins et al., 2016; Slade et al., 2018). This approach can enhance patient satisfaction, improve adherence to treatment plans and promote a sense of ownership over their healthcare journey.

In Chinese contexts, where family involvement in healthcare decision-making is culturally significant, involving patients and their families in handovers may be particularly beneficial. Families in China often play a key role in managing the healthcare of their relatives, and their inclusion in the handover process can lead to more informed decisions and better support for the patient (Pun et al., 2018). However, there are also challenges to consider. Some nurses may feel uncomfortable involving patients in handovers, particularly when discussing sensitive medical information or potential risks. Additionally, cultural norms of deference to authority may make patients hesitant to ask questions or challenge the information presented during handovers, limiting their engagement in the process (Pun, 2023a). To overcome these challenges, hospitals should provide guidance on how to effectively involve patients in handovers while maintaining professionalism and confidentiality. Nurses should be trained to create a welcoming environment where patients and families feel comfortable participating, while also ensuring that medical terminology is explained in a way that is easily understandable.

*

Communication during nursing handovers is a critical determinant of patient safety and the seamless continuity of care. As one of the most pivotal points in the patient care process, the quality of information exchanged during handovers directly impacts patient outcomes, particularly in high-pressure environments like hospitals. In the Chinese contexts, however, effective communication during handover is often complicated by hierarchical relationship and cultural norms that can discourage open dialogue and limit the flow of critical information. The deeply ingrained respect for authority, combined with the cultural emphasis on maintaining harmony and avoiding conflict, can create an environment where junior nurses feel hesitant to seek clarification or raise concerns, even when doing so is essential for patient safety. These cultural and organisational barriers must be carefully navigated to ensure that handovers are conducted effectively. Despite these challenges, the use of structured communication tools like ISBAR offers a clear and practical solution. ISBAR provides a standardised framework that ensures all relevant information is conveyed systematically, reducing the potential for misunderstandings or omissions. This structured approach is particularly valuable in hierarchical settings, as it provides a formal mechanism for asking questions and seeking clarification, thereby normalising behaviours that might otherwise be constrained by cultural factors. While ISBAR offers structure, its effectiveness can be limited by language proficiency and ingrained hierarchical barriers, particularly among junior staff.

The role of clinicians in this process cannot be overstated. Clinicians, as both educators and role models, are uniquely positioned to help nurses develop the skills and confidence necessary to navigate the complexities of handover communication. Through comprehensive training programmes, clinicians can teach nurses not only how to use structured communication tools effectively but also how to engage in meaningful, two-way communication. These programmes should prioritise the development of interpersonal communication skills, such as active listening, asking clarifying questions and providing feedback, which are crucial for ensuring mutual understanding during handovers. Additionally, clinicians should foster a supportive environment that encourages nurses to challenge hierarchical norms and assert their voices in the interest of patient safety. This includes creating safe spaces for practice, such as role-playing and simulation exercises, where nurses can build the confidence to communicate effectively in real-world settings.

Furthermore, training programmes should address the realities of high patient loads and time pressures that often characterise hospital environments in China. Nurses need to be equipped with strategies for conducting efficient yet thorough handovers, where the most critical information is prioritised and clearly communicated within limited timeframes. By teaching nurses how to manage these competing demands, clinicians can help ensure that handovers are not rushed or incomplete, even in the most challenging of circumstances. The ultimate goal of these training efforts is to cultivate a culture of open communication, where all nurses feel empowered to contribute actively to the handover process, regardless of their rank or experience. To conclude, the quality of nursing handovers can be significantly improved through a combination of structured communication protocols, targeted training and a cultural shift towards open dialogue and interaction. By addressing the unique challenges posed by hierarchical structures and cultural norms in the Chinese context, clinicians can play a transformative role in enhancing the effectiveness of handovers. Through these efforts, the safety, efficiency and continuity of patient care can be greatly improved, leading to better outcomes for both patients and healthcare providers. In an increasingly complex and fast-paced healthcare environment, fostering high-quality communication during nursing handovers is not just a best practice – it is a necessity for ensuring the highest standards of patient care and safety.

To conclude, effective communication during nursing handovers is a critical component of patient safety and continuity of care. This chapter has examined the complex interplay of cultural norms, hierarchical structures and institutional constraints that shape handover practices in Chinese healthcare settings. The discussion highlighted key challenges, such as junior nurses' reluctance to speak up, time pressures and language barriers, which can all contribute to communication breakdowns. To address these issues, structured communication frameworks such as ISBAR have been identified as effective tools for standardising handover processes, ensuring clarity and promoting patient safety. However, while structured protocols provide a useful foundation, they must be complemented by training in interpersonal communication skills, active listening and fostering a culture of open dialogue. By empowering nurses with the necessary skills and confidence to engage actively in handovers, healthcare institutions can improve the accuracy and effectiveness of information exchange, ultimately enhancing patient outcomes.

As healthcare settings in Hong Kong and other Chinese contexts continue to evolve, it is imperative to develop culturally informed handover strategies that acknowledge both traditional hierarchical norms and the growing emphasis on patient-centred care. Future research should further explore the role of multilingualism, digital tools and patient involvement in optimising handover communication. By bridging the gap between standardised protocols and the realities of clinical practice, healthcare systems can work towards a more resilient and communicatively competent nursing workforce.

Building on the discussion of nursing communication, the next chapter shifts focus to broader medical communication strategies across clinical disciplines in Hong Kong. The next conclusing chapter synthesises key findings from previous discussions, offering policy recommendations for developing culturally appropriate communication models. By critically examining clinician-patient interactions, multilingual dynamics and the impact of cultural values on medical discourse, the next section provides insights into the future directions of healthcare communication research and practice in the region.

13

Conclusion, discussion and policy recommendations

Overviewing the last twelve chapters in general and discipline-specific clinical contexts unique to East Asian settings and Hong Kong, it is significant for researchers and clinicians to be culturally competent in order to design appropriate communication models instead of directly adopting Western models. For example, clinicians in Hong Kong code-switch or perform translanguaging with other doctors and nurses in spoken Cantonese as well as English medical terms. A lack of research has been conducted to understand how that has affected the effectiveness of communication in different areas, which is why more research is needed to develop appropriate frameworks. By employing knowledge from applied linguistics and medical communication, we included primary data from interviews with surgeons, neurologists, oncologists, ED and ICU clinicians as well as geriatricians in Hong Kong. These insights have addressed the key themes identified by the author as unique to Chinese and other East Asian contexts, including power and relationships among healthcare providers, patients and families; cultural attitudes and communication preferences affecting trust, decision-making and patient satisfaction; Chinese model of patient-centred care; and the rise of health literacy of patients. This concluding chapter summarises the list of communication strategies for promoting effective clinical communication in Hong Kong and then advocates an agenda to study Chinese cultural elements closely when designing effective clinical communication for clinicians and researchers to learn how patients, their carers and healthcare providers reflect on their practices.

Characteristics of medical communication in East Asian settings and Hong Kong

Many previous research projects have neglected the cultural aspects of communication in medical settings (Pun et al., 2018). Noting such a research gap, we have unveiled the reasons behind East Asian patients being unwilling to ask direct questions or speak about their concerns in high-context cultures like Japan, South Korea and China (Pun et al., 2018). We included the primary findings from local clinicians in Hong Kong that showed how collectivist and individualist values form Asian healthcare contexts, especially in relation to multilingual cultural settings like Hong Kong and Singapore. Moreover, the insights reported in the previous chapters reflected a tendency for patients to shift from collectivist beliefs to higher recognition of patient autonomy in Hong Kong, Singapore and Taiwan. Therefore, the key goal of clinicians when implementing patient-centred care should be encouraging their patients to participate as informed stakeholders and feel respected by acknowledging their individual preferences, needs and beliefs (Slade et al., 2015a). It appears that there is still a huge gap between theory and real-life practice in the implementation of patient-centred policies, calling for the need for attention from practitioners and hospitals.

Implementing culturally appropriate patient-centred care in East Asia

As noted, it is important for practitioners and hospitals to consider the cultural norms and backgrounds of the respective cultures. For instance, patients' families in Asia usually play a key role when making shared medical decisions. This shows the varying power and relationship dynamics between Asian and the dualist Western communication framework of clinician-patient conversations (Pun et al., 2018). While a number of research projects showed that Asian patients in general prefer their doctors to be more dominant in a paternalistic and asymmetrical style during medical discussions, recent studies have discovered that some desire to be more active when making decisions (Pun et al., 2018). Moreover, clinicians in East Asia tend to prioritise medical topics over interpersonal matters. Although some East Asian patients accept such an approach due to the level of respect they have for their physicians' professional expertise, they also like to communicate their wishes during decision-making processes (Pun et al., 2018). The findings included in the previous chapters resonated with Claramaita et al.'s (2013) research, which demonstrated the tension in Asian settings between a tendency to adopt Western patient-centred communication frameworks and advocate patient autonomy while respecting local cultures that might be incompatible with the values inherent in existing models (Pun et al., 2018). Therefore, we have integrated first-hand insights from local clinicians from different disciplines in Hong Kong in order to understand the value of the Western patient-centred communication frameworks and learn how they could be carefully adapted to fit the local context (Pun et al., 2016). In addition, we have proved that patients who actively participate in decision-making processes tend to show higher levels of patient satisfaction regardless of the cultural differences in their preferred degrees of decision-making and patient autonomy across various Asian regions (Boon & Stewart, 1998). Extending on such findings, the previous chapters have offered a guidance for future researchers to design further studies to learn about the relationships between patient involvement, the quality of their patients' care and safety.

According to the last twelve chapters, some key themes in healthcare communication in East Asian contexts and particularly Hong Kong have emerged, namely (1) clinicians' prioritisation of patients' physical comfort over psycho-emotional needs; (2) hierarchical and asymmetrical interactions between physicians and patients; (3) the tension between the dominant role of patients' families and patient autonomy; (4) an urgency for clinicians to develop cultural competence and apply cultural knowledge in real-life settings; (5) challenges for clinicians to carry out difficult conversations like EOL matters due to taboo subjects like death; (6) different communication preferences across various East Asian regions that affect trust, the processes of decision-making and patient satisfaction; (7) clinicians' observations of cultural preferences and dynamics as well as non-verbal language in multicultural settings (Pun et al., 2018). In the latter sections, we review how the findings from the previous chapters have reflected the stated observations and recommend research frameworks for future researchers to consider when exploring the role of healthcare interactions in Asia and Hong Kong.

Discipline-specific tactics for communication: Researching the multilingual clinical contexts of Hong Kong through interviews

By employing interdisciplinary approaches to the investigation of medical communication in East Asian contexts and integrating methodologies widely used in applied linguistics, we have generated new discoveries from existing studies and original interview transcripts across disciplines. Such approaches have enabled the involved researchers to unveil the complexity and unique aspects of specific medical settings, including surgery, neurology, oncology, nursing, palliative care, ICU and geriatric in the trilingual environment of Hong Kong. Chapters 3 to 12 have demonstrated step-by-step guides for researchers to design discipline-specific qualitative studies in cross-cultural clinical environments while considering quantitative data from former studies. The chapters have also emphasised the importance of interdisciplinary understanding in the pursuit of understanding how multicultural elements affect the nature of communication case-by-case.

Solving hierarchy in clinician-to-clinician relationships across disciplines in Hong Kong

As noted, hierarchies are often observed in East Asian and Chinese medical contexts. Therefore, to accommodate Chinese Confucian cultural beliefs like ensuring harmony and preventing conflicts, Asia-based clinicians tend to use certain recurring communication strategies. For instance, ICU nurses and doctors with different ranks would have varying perceptions of speaking up. It is suggested that ICU clinicians should speak up both within their unit and across other medical departments as the ICU is interdisciplinary in nature. To accomplish that, individual clinicians and the hospital should facilitate communication by endorsing the value of promoting respect and communication openness. Clinicians need to be trained to speak freely considering the influences of Chinese Confucian values in Hong Kong and other Chinese settings. Human factors and values should be stressed over conflict management in East Asian medical contexts.

The power dynamics between patients and their families: The influences of collectivist and individualist values in Hong Kong

We have explored the tension between collectivist and individualist values in some East Asian contexts, including Taiwan, Singapore and particularly Hong Kong. Due to the prevailing influence of the collectivist family-centred attitude in Chinese EOL conversations (Sun et al., 2011), many patients have been unable to learn about factual information about their conditions as their families hide such information from them due to cultural taboos (Zheng et al., 2015; Wong-Kim et al., 2003). As a result, patients are sometimes unable to make informed decisions as patient autonomy is hindered. Therefore, clinicians need to learn to strike a balance between fulfilling patients' familial needs and their autonomy. They are advised to foster (1) medical discussions between patients and clinicians; (2) patients' interactions with their relatives, which allow the latter to offer advice and comfort; (3) patients' voicing of their requests and plans; (4) patients' expressions of their feelings and personal thoughts on treatments. For instance, MV patients in Hong Kong's ICU settings want to be part of discussions about their conditions with their clinicians, showing traces of individualist values. At the same time, they want to connect with their family members to seek and offer support to fulfil psycho-emotional needs. Neurologists also often have to be capable of managing both their patients and families' expectations, considering a lot of neurological issues require them to seek realistic forms of hope in rather grim situations (Clayton et al., 2007). Neurologists, geriatricians, ED and ICU clinicians also often have to communicate mainly with relatives when patients are unconscious, making it extremely crucial for them to make the families feel that they are empathetic, doing their best and willing to improve their health literacy (Zehm et al., 2020). In short, clinicians need to carefully observe the power dynamics in their patients' familial relations when individualism and Confucianism merge together in Hong Kong.

A guide for local practitioners: Tailoring difficult conversations according to cultural backgrounds

The recurring theme of the taboo subject of death and the idea of a 'good death' has been emphasised throughout the book. Due to the presence of such a taboo, a lot of clinicians across disciplines tend to find it hard for them to deliver bad news as Asian patients have varying perceptions towards EOL discussions when compared to the West or even other East Asian settings. Interestingly, geriatricians in Hong Kong have observed that many of their patients are more positive towards ACP and AD, contrary to the common belief of all Asian patients shying away from such topics. To cater to different patients' attitudes towards EOL matters, it is recommended that clinicians teach their juniors by applying virtual reality simulators and setting up role-play sessions in order for them to learn to be culturally sensitive and about family-oriented approaches to EOL communication.

When training medical professionals and students for EOL communication, researchers are encouraged to design programmes that educate students to be attentive to their patients' emotional and cultural needs, respect their relatives' wishes during decision-making processes, make use of indirect communication strategies when delivering shocking news and help fulfil the patients' familial needs. In addition to that, although many studies have claimed that most Asian patients tend to be greatly influenced by collectivist values, many from Hong Kong, Taiwan and Singapore have a strong desire for their individual thoughts to be listened to and respected. Thus, it is crucial for researchers to design culturally appropriate communication models in order to teach healthcare professionals what a 'good death' is in relevant cultural contexts such as Confucian, Taoist and/or Buddhist beliefs, which would in turn help them manage their patients and relatives' negative perceptions towards EOL discussions and carry out open conversations.

How to build rapport between practitioners and patients in Hong Kong

A lot of patients in Hong Kong consult TCM practitioners in addition to WM in Hong Kong (Chung et al., 2009). It is worthwhile for Hong Kong-based doctors to consider how their TCM counterparts' holistic approaches to clinician-patient communication offer insights into ways to achieve improved patient understanding and compliance with preferred treatment plans (Pun, 2020a; 2020b; 2020c; 2020d). Instead of merely focusing on treating physical symptoms, doctors are encouraged to also help their patients heal. TCM practitioners evaluate many aspects of the patients' personal life, body conditions as well as outer environments (Chan, 1995; Zhou & Nunes, 2012) using the four methods of wàng望 (look), wén聞 (Listen and smell), wèn問 (Question) and qiè切 (Pulse-diagnosis). This enables TCM practitioners to take care of their patients' therapeutic care through medical and interpersonal perspectives, and eventually deliver patient-centred care. It would be invaluable for WM doctors to learn how TCM practitioners show better communication abilities through listening to their patients' opinions, leading them to share information regarding their personal lives as well as healthcare issues, responding timely and appropriately, being understanding, asking questions with caution in order to build trusting yet professional relationships with the patients and acknowledging the significant role of small talk. These insights could be integrated into communication training programmes for WM practitioners, so they can develop skills for forming good doctor-patient relationships in the cultural settings of Hong Kong and other Chinese societies.

To conclude, we have unveiled significant insights into the multicultural and multilingual dynamics of healthcare communication in Hong Kong. In an increasingly diverse society, effective clinical communication is not just about language proficiency – it is about cultural competence, empathy and the ability to adapt communication strategies to meet the needs of a wide range of patients. The challenges faced by ethnic minorities in accessing equitable healthcare highlight the urgent need for clinicians to develop skills beyond traditional verbal interactions. Understanding non-verbal cues, utilising visual aids and integrating professional translation services can bridge the communication gap and foster more inclusive healthcare environments.

Moving forward, there is a critical need for interdisciplinary research that explores how multilingual and multicultural communication impacts patient safety, trust and treatment adherence. Future studies could investigate the effectiveness of digital translation tools in real-time clinical interactions, explore best practices for incorporating culturally appropriate communication training into medical education and examine the role of family dynamics in decision-making within diverse patient populations. Additionally, as Hong Kong's healthcare system continues to integrate advanced technologies, research on AI-assisted communication tools and their ethical implications in clinical settings will be crucial.

Ultimately, the findings presented in this book reinforce the importance of a patient-centred approach to medical communication – one that respects linguistic diversity, cultural identities and individual healthcare needs. By fostering a more inclusive and culturally competent healthcare system, clinicians can improve patient experiences, reduce disparities and enhance the overall quality of care. The journey towards better clinical communication does not end here; rather, it opens new avenues for research, policy development and training initiatives that will shape the future of healthcare communication in Hong Kong and beyond.

References

Abbey, J. G. (2008). *Communication about end-of-life topics between terminally ill cancer patients and their family members* (Doctoral dissertation, ETD Collection for Fordham University).

Adams, C. L., & Kurtz, S. M. (2017). *Skills for communicating in veterinary medicine.* Otmoor Publishing.

Afriyie, D. (2020). Effective communication between nurses and patients: An evolutionary concept analysis. *British Journal of Community Nursing, 25*(9), 438–445.

Ahalt, C., Walter, L. C., Yourman, L., Eng, C., Perez-Stable, E. J., & Smith, A. K. (2012). "Knowing is better": Preferences of diverse older adults for discussing prognosis. *Journal of General Internal Medicine*, 27, 568–575.

Aita, V., McIlvain, H., Backer, E., McVea, K., & Crabtree, B. (2005). Patient-centered care and communication in primary care practice: What is involved? *Patient Education and Counseling, 58*(3), 296–304.

Alegrıa, M., Sribney, W., Perez, D., Laderman, M., & Keefe, K. (2009). The role of patient activation on patient–provider communication and quality of care for US and foreign-born Latino patients. *Journal of General Internal Medicine, 24*, 534–541.

Ali, P. A., & Johnson, S. (2017). Speaking my patient's language: Bilingual nurses' perspective about provision of language concordant care to patients with limited English proficiency. *Journal of Advanced Nursing, 73*(2), 421–432.

Almack, K., Cox, K., Moghaddam, N., et al. (2012). After you: Conversations between patients and healthcare professionals in planning for end of life care. *BMC Palliative Care, 11*, 15.

Al Shamsi, H., Almutairi, A. G., Al Mashrafi, S., & Al Kalbani, T. (2020). Implications of language barriers for healthcare: A systematic review. *Oman Medical Journal, 35*(2), e122.

Al-Shura, A. N. (2014). Patient perspectives. In Anika Niambi Al-Shura (ed.), *Integrative cardiovascular Chinese medicine: A prevention and personalized medicine perspective* (pp. 39–56). Elsevier Academic Press.

Amutio-Kareaga, A., García-Campayo, J., Delgado, L. C., Hermosilla, D., & Martínez-Taboada, C. (2017). Improving communication between physicians and their patients through mindfulness and compassion-based strategies: A narrative review. *Journal of Clinical Medicine, 6*(3), 33.

Anderson, J., Malone, L., Shanahan, K., & Manning, J. (2015). Nursing bedside clinical handover–an integrated review of issues and tools. *Journal of Clinical Nursing, 24*(5–6), 662–671.

Andersson, E. K., Willman, A., Sjöström-Strand, A., & Borglin, G. (2014). Registered nurses' descriptions of caring: A phenomenographic interview study. *BMC Nursing, 14*, 16.

Anestis, E., Eccles, F. J. R., Fletcher, I., & Simpson, J. (2021). Neurologists' current practice and perspectives on communicating the diagnosis of a motor neurodegenerative condition: A UK survey. *BMC Neurology, 21*(34), e1–9.

Angelelli, C. V. (2004). *Medical interpreting and cross-cultural communication.* Cambridge University Press.

Apker, J., Mallak, L. A., & Gibson, S. C. (2007). Communicating in the "Gray Zone": Perceptions about Emergency Physician–hospitalist Handoffs and Patient Safety. *Academic Emergency Medicine, 14*, 884–894.

Arsenault, M., Long, S., D'Souza, V., Ilie, A., & Todd, K. J. (2024). Telemedicine visits requiring follow-up in-person visits at an urban academic family medicine centre. *Family Practice, 41*(2), 105–113.

Artemiou, E., Adams, C. L., Hecker, K. G., Vallevand, A., Violato, C., & Coe, J. B. (2014). Standardised clients as assessors in a veterinary communication OSCE: A reliability and validity study. *Veterinary Record, 175*, 509.

Arthur, D., Chong, C., Rujkorakarn, D., Wong, D., & Wongpanarak, N. (2004). A profile of the caring attributes of Hong Kong and Thailand psychiatric nurses. *International Journal of Mental Health Nursing, 13*(2), 100–106.

Ashworth, P. (Eds.). (1980). *Care to communicate: An investigation into problems of communication between patients and nurses in intensive therapy units.* Royal College of Nursing of UK Research Series. Whitefriars Press.

Attree, M. (2001). Patients' and relatives' experiences and perspectives of 'good' and 'not so good' quality care. *Journal of Advanced Nursery, 33*(4), 456–466.

Ayoko, O. B. (2007). Communication openness, conflict events and reactions to conflict in culturally diverse workgroups. *Cross Cultural Management: An International Journal, 14*, 105–24.

Ayonrinde, O. (2003). Importance of cultural sensitivity in therapeutic transactions. *Disease Management & Health Outcomes, 11*, 233–2483.

Baile, W. F., Buckman, R., Lenzi, R., Glober, G., Beale, E. A., & Kudelka, A. P. (2000). SPIKES—a six-step protocol for delivering bad news: application to the patient with cancer. *The oncologist*, 5(4), 302–311.

Ballantyne, K. C., & Buller, K. (2015). Experiences of veterinarians in clinical behavior practice: A mixed-methods study. *Journal of Veterinary Behaviour: Clinical Applications and Research, 10*(5), 376–383.

Barclay, J. S., Blackhall, L. J., & Tulsky, J. A. (2007). Communication strategies and cultural issues in the delivery of bad news. *Journal of Palliative Medicine, 10*(4), 958–977.

Barwise, A. (2019). *End of life care and decision making for patients with limited English* proficiency (Doctoral dissertation, College of Medicine-Mayo Clinic).

Barwise, A., Jaramillo, C., Novotny, P., et al. (2018). Differences in code status and end-of-life decision making in patients with limited English proficiency in the intensive care unit. *Mayo Clinic Proceedings, 93*(9), 1271–1281.

Bazargan, M., & Bazargan-Hejazi, S. (2021). Disparities in palliative and hospice care and completion of advance care planning and directives among non-Hispanic blacks: A scoping review of recent literature. *American Journal of Hospice and Palliative Medicine, 38*, 688–718.

Bazargan, M., Cobb, S., Assari, S., & Kibe, L. W. (2021). Awareness of palliative care, hospice care, and advance directives in a racially and ethnically diverse sample of California adults. *American Journal of Hospice and Palliative Medicine, 38*, 601–9.

Beach, W. A. (2015). Doctor-patient interaction. In K. Tracy (Ed.), *Encyclopedia of language and social interaction* (pp. 476–493). John Wiley & Sons, Inc.

Beisecker, A. E. (1990). Patient power in doctor-patient communication: What do we know? *Health Communication, 2*(2), 105–122.

Bergbom-Engberg, I. H. H. (1989). Assessment of patients' experience of discomforts during respiratory therapy. *Critical Care Medicine, 17*(10), 1068–1072.

Berkman, N. D., Sheridan, S. L., Donahue, K. E., et al. (2011). Health literacy interventions and outcomes: An updated systematic review. *Evidence Report Technology Assessment, 199*, 1–941.

Betancourt, J. (2006). Cultural competency: Providing quality care to diverse populations. *The Consultant Pharmacist, 21*(12), 988–995.

Bezemer, J., Cope, A., Korkiakangas, T., et al. (2017). Microanalysis of video from the operating room: An underused approach to patient safety research. *BMJ Quality & Safety, 26*, 583–587.

Bischoff, A., Perneger, T. V., Bovier, P. A., Lou-tan, L., & Stalder, H. (2003). Improving communication between physicians and patients who speak a foreign language. *British Journal of General Practice, 53*, 541–546.

Boersma, I., Miyasaki, J., Kutner, J., & Kluger, B. (2014). Palliative care and neurology: Time for a paradigm shift. *Neurology, 83*, 561–567.

Bouhdili, N. (2015). *How pulse diagnosis works by transformational acupuncture.* Available at https://www.dc-acupuncture.com/physical-health/how-pulsediagnosis-works.

Bourhis, R., Roth, S., & Macqueen, G. (1989). Communication in the hospital setting: A survey of medical and everyday language use amongst patients, nurses and doctors. *Social Science & Medicine, 28*, 339–346.

Bowling, A., Rowe, G., & McKee, M. (2013). Patients' experiences of their healthcare in relation to their expectations and satisfaction: A population survey. *Journal of the Royal Society of Medicine, 106*(4), 143–149.

Bowman, F. M., Goldberg, D. P., Millar, T., Gask, L., & Mcgrath, G. (1992). Improving the skills of established general practitioners: The long-term benefits of group teaching. *Medical Education, 26*(1), 63–68.

Bowman, K. W., & Singer, P. A. (2001). Chinese seniors' perspectives on end-of-life decisions. *Social Science & Medicine (1982), 53*(4), 455–464.

Boyd, K. (2001). Deciding about resuscitation. *Journal of Medical Ethics, 27*(5), 291–294.

Brooks, T. R. (1992). Pitfalls in communication with Hispanic and African-American patients: Do translators help or harm? *Journal of the National Medical Association, 84*, 941.

Broyles, L. M., Tate, J. A., & Happ, M. B. (2012). Use of augmentative and alternative communication strategies by family members in the intensive care unit. *American Journal of Critical Care, 21*(2), e21–e22.

Bruton, J., Norton, C., Smyth, N., Ward, H., & Day, S. (2016). Nurse handover: Patient and staff experiences. *British Journal of Nursing, 25*(7), 386–393.

Burckhardt, C. S. (2005). Educating patients: Self-management approaches. *Disability and Rehabilitation, 27*(12), 703–709.

Burgess, A., Van Diggele, C., Roberts, C., & Mellis, C. (2020). Teaching clinical handover with ISBAR. *BMC Medical Education, 20*, 1–8.

Car, J., Tan, W. S., Huang, Z., Sloot, P., & Franklin, B. D. (2017). eHealth in the future of medications management: Personalisation, monitoring and adherence. *BMC Medicine, 15*, 1–9.

Carrillo, J. E., Green, A. R., & Betancourt, J. R. (1999). Cross-cultural primary care: A patient-based approach. *Annals of Internal Medicine, 130*(10), 829–834.

Carroll, S. M. (2004). Nonvocal ventilated patients perceptions of being understood. *Western Journal of Nursing Research, 26*(1), 85–103.

Carroll, S. M. (2007). Silent, slow lifeworld: The communication experience of nonvocal ventilated patients. *Qualitative Health Research, 17*(9), 1165–1677.

Carter, M., Thompson, N., Crampton, P., Morrow, G., Burford, B., Gray, C., & Illing, J. (2013). Workplace bullying in the UK NHS: A questionnaire and interview study on prevalence, impact and barriers to reporting. *BMJ Open, 3*, e002628.

Carver, A. C., Vickrey, B. G., Bernat, J. L., Keran, C., Ringel, S. P., & Foley, K. M. (1999). End-of-life care: A survey of US neurologists' attitudes, behavior, and knowledge. *Neurology, 53*, 284–293.

Chan, A., & Woodruff, R. K. (1999). Comparison of palliative care needs of English- and non-English-speaking patients. *Journal of Palliative Care, 15*(1), 26–30.

Chan, C. L. W., Tsuji-Abe, Y., & Chan, T. H. Y. (2006). What is good death: Bridging the gap between research and intervention. In Chan C. L. W. & Chow A. Y. M. (Eds.), *Death, dying and bereavement: A Hong Kong Chinese experience* (p. 127). Hong Kong University Press.

Chan, E. A. (2011). Nurses' perception of time availability in patient communication in Hong Kong. *Journal of Clinical Nursing, 21*(7–8), 1168–1177.

Chan, H. Y., & Pang, S. M. (2007). Quality of life concerns and end-of-life care preferences of aged persons in long-term care facilities. *Journal of Clinical Nursing, 16*(11), 2158–2166.

Chan, J. C. Y., Gupta, A. K., Stewart, S., Babidge, W., McCulloch, G., Worthington, M. G., & Maddern, G. J. (2019). "Nobody told me": Communication issues affecting australian cardiothoracic surgery patients. *The Annals of Thoracic Surgery, 108(*6), 1801–1806.

Chan, K. (1995). Progress in traditional Chinese medicine. *Trends in Pharmacological Sciences, 16*(6), 182–187.

Chan, W. C. H. (2011). Being aware of the prognosis: How does it relate to palliative care patients' anxiety and communication difficulty with family members in the Hong Kong Chinese context? *Journal of Palliative Medicine, 14*(9), 997–1003.

Chan, E. A., Jones, A., Fung, S., & Wu, S. C. (2012). Nurses' perception of time availability in patient communication in Hong Kong. *Journal of clinical nursing,* 21(7–8), 1168–1177.

Chan, C. M. H., Ahmad, W. A. W., Yusof, M., Ho, G. F., & Krupat, E. (2015). Patient-centredness, job satisfaction and psychological distress: a brief survey comparing oncology nurses and doctors. *Asian Pacific Journal of Cancer Prevention,* 16(16), 6895–6898.

Chandler, E., Slade, D., Pun, J., Lock, G., Matthiessen, C. M. I. M., Espindola, E., & Ng, C. (2015). Communication in Hong Kong accident & emergency departments: The clinicians' perspectives. *Global Qualitative Nursing Journal, 2,* 1–11.

Charles, C., Gafni, A., & Whelan, T. (1999). Decision-making in the physician–patient encounter: Revisiting the shared treatment decision-making model. *Social Science & Medicine, 49*(5), 651–661.

Chen, D., Jerng, J., Tsai, D. F., & Young, Y. (2022). Gender differences in the intention to withhold life-sustaining treatments involving severe dementia for self and on behalf of parent or spouse. *BMC Palliative Care, 21,* 1–12.

Chen, D., & Weng, H. (2023). Associations of health literacy, personality traits, and pro-individualism with the willingness to complete advance directives in Taiwan. *BMC Palliative Care, 22*(91), 1–14.

Cherniack, E. P. (2002). Increasing use of DNR orders in the elderly worldwide: Whose choice is it? *Journal of Medical Ethics, 28*(5), 303–307.

Cheung, D. S., Kelly, J. J., Beach, C., et al. (2010). Improving handoffs in the emergency department. *Annals of Emergency Medicine, 55*(2), 171–180.

Chewning, B., Bylund, C., Shah, B., Arora, N. K., Gueguen, J. A., & Makoul, G. (2012). Patient preferences for shared decisions: A systematic review. *Patient Education and Counseling, 86,* 9–18.

Chi, H., Cataldo, J., Ho, E. Y., & Rehm, R. S. (2018). Please ask gently: Using culturally targeted communication strategies to initiate end-of-life care discussions with older Chinese Americans. *American Journal of Hospice and Palliative Medicine, 35*(10), 1265–1272.

Chien, L. J., Slade, D., Dahm, M. R., Brady, B., Roberts, E., Goncharov, L., ... & Thornton, A. (2022). Improving patient-centred care through a tailored intervention addressing nursing clinical handover communication in its organizational and cultural context. *Journal of Advanced Nursing, 78*(5), 1413–1430.

Chiò, A., Montuschi, A., Cammarosano, S., De Mercanti, S., Cavallo, E., Ilardi, A., Ghiglione, P., Mutani, R., & Calvo, A. (2008). ALS patients and caregivers communication preferences and information seeking behaviour. *European Journal of Neurology, 15*, 55–60.

Chisholm, C. D., Collison, E. K., Nelson, D. R., & Cordell, W. H. (2000). Emergency department workplace interruptions: Are emergency physicians "interrupt-driven" and "multitasking"? *Academic Emergency Medicine, 7*, 1239–1243.

Christ, M., Schuh, K., & Bayas, A. (2023). Large-scale cross-sectional online survey on patient-neurologist communication, burden of disease assessment and disease monitoring in people with multiple sclerosis. *Frontiers in Neurology, 13*, e1–e13.

Christakis, N. A. (1999). *Death foretold: Prophecy and prognosis in medical care.* University of Chicago Press.

Christakis, N. A., & Iwashyna, T. J. (1998). Attitude and self-reported practice regarding prognostication in a national sample of internists. *Archives of Internal Medicine, 158*, 2389–2395.

Chu, W., & Woo, J. (2004). Attitudes of Chinese elders towards advance planning on end-of-life issues: A qualitative study in a nursing home in Hong Kong. *Journal of the Hong Kong Geriatrics Society, 12*(1), 18–23.

Chung, J. Y. S., Li, W. H. C., Cheung, A. T., Ho, L. L. K., & Chung, J. O. K. (2022). Efficacy of a blended learning programme in enhancing the communication skill competence and self-efficacy of nursing students in conducting clinical handovers: A randomised controlled trial. *BMC Medical Education, 22*(1), 275.

Chung, V. C. H., Lau, C. H., Wong, E. M., Yeoh, E. K., & Griffiths, S. M. (2009). Perceived quality of communication amongst outpatients in western and traditional Chinese medicine clinics in a Chinese population. *Health Policy (New York), 90*(1), 66–72.

Claramita, M., Nugraheni, M. D., van Dalen, J., & Vleuten, C. van der. (2013). Doctor–patient communication in Southeast Asia: A different culture? *Advances in Health Sciences Education, 18*(1), 15–31.

Claramita, M., & Susilo, A. P. (2014). Improving communication skills in the Southeast Asian health care context. *Perspectives on Medical Education, 3*(6), 474–479.

Clark, P. G. (1995). Quality of life, values, and teamwork in geriatric care: Do we communicate what we mean? *The Gerontologist, 35*(3), 402–411.

Clarke, V., & Braun, V. (2014). Thematic analysis. In T. Teo (Ed.), *Encyclopedia of critical psychology* (pp. 1947–1952). Springer.

Clayman, M. L., Roter, D., Wissow, L. S., et al. (2005). Autonomy-related behaviors of patient companions and their effect on decision-making activity in geriatric primary care visits. *Social Science & Medicine, 60*, 1583–1591.

Clayton, J. M., Hancock, K. M., Butow, P. N., et al. (2007). Clinical practice guidelines for communicating prognosis and end-of-life issues with adults in the advanced stages of a life-limiting illness, and their caregivers. *Medical Journal of Australia, 186*(12 suppl), S77, S79, S83–108.

Coiera, E., Jayasuriya, R., Hardy, J., & Thrope, M. E. (2002). Communication loads on clinical staff in the emergency department. *Medical Journal of Australia, 176*, 415–418.

Cong, Y. (2004). Doctor-family-patient relationship: The Chinese paradigm of informed consent. *The Journal of Medicine and Philosophy, 29*(2), 149–178.

Creutzfeldt, C. J., Robinson, M. T., & Holloway, R. G. (2016). Neurologists as primary palliative care providers: Communication and practice approaches. *Neurology Clinical Practice, 6*, 40–48.

Creutzfeldt, C., Gooley, T., & Walker, M. (2009). Are neurology residents prepared to deal with dying patients? *Archives of Neurology, 66*, 1427–1428.

Cui, J., Shen, F., Ma, X., & Zhao, J. (2011). What do nurses want to learn from death education? A survey of their needs. *Oncology Nursing Forum, 38*(6), E402–e408.

Cumin, D., Skilton, C., & Weller, J. (2016). Information transfer in multidisciplinary operating room teams: A simulation-based observational study. *BMJ Quality and Safety, 26*, 209–216.

Dahm, M. R. (2011). Exploring perception and use of everyday language and medical terminology among international medical graduates in a medical ESP course in Australia. *English for Specific Purpose, 30*, 186–197.

Dahm, M. R. (2012). Coming to terms with medical terms–exploring insights from native and non-native English speakers in patient-physician communication. *Hermes Journal Language of Communication Business, 25*, 79.

Dallara, A., Meret, A., & Saryan, J. (2014). Mapping the literature: Palliative care within adult and child neurology. *Journal of Child Neurology, 29*, 1728–1738.

Dang, B. N., Westbrook, R. A., Njue, S. M., & Giordano, T. P. (2017). Building trust and rapport early in the new doctor-patient relationship: A longitudinal qualitative study. *BMC Medical Education, 17*, 1–10.

De Boer, M. E., Dröes, R-M., Jonker, C., Eefsting, J. A., & Hertogh, C. M. P. M. (2012). Thoughts on the future: The perspectives of elderly people with early-stage Alzheimer's disease and the implications for advance care planning. *AJOB Primary Research, 3*, 14–22.

Deep, K. S., Griffith, C. H., & Wilson, J. F. (2008). Discussing preferences for cardiopulmonary resuscitation: What do resident physicians and their hospitalized patients think was decided? *Patient Education and Counseling, 72*(1), 20–25.

Deledda, G., Moretti, F., Rimondini, M., & Zimmermann, C. (2013). How patients want their doctor to communicate. A literature review on primary care patients' perspective. *Patient Education and Counseling, 90*(3), 297–306.

Demjén, Zsófia. *Applying linguistics in illness and healthcare contexts*. Bloomsbury.

Dening, K. H., Jones, L., & Sampson, E. L. (2011). Advance care planning for people with dementia: A review. *International Psychogeriatrics, 23*, 1535–1551.

Desmond, J., & Copeland, L. R. (2000). *Communicating with today's patient: Essentials to save time, decrease risk, and increase patient compliance*. John Wiley & Sons.

Diamond, L., Chung, S., Ferguson, W., et al. (2014). Relationship between self-assessed and tested non–English-language proficiency among primary care providers. *Med Care, 52*(5), 435–438.

Dias, L., Chabner, B. A., Lynch, T. J., & Penson, R. T. (2003). Breaking bad news: A patient's perspective. *Oncologist, 8*(6), 587–596.

Dickinson, G. E., Roof, P. D., & Roof, K. W. (2011). A survey of veterinarians in the US: Euthanasia and other end-of-life issues. *Anthrozoos, 24*, 167–174.

Dong, F., & Yin, M. (2012). The strategy of telling the true diagnostic information to cancer patient. *The Journal of Medicine and Philosophy, 33*, 666–668.

Dong, F., Zheng, R., Chen, X., Wang, Y., Zhou, H., & Sun, R. (2016). Caring for dying cancer patients in the Chinese cultural context: A qualitative study from the perspectives of physicians and nurses. *European Journal of Oncology Nursing, 21*, 189–196.

Douglas, M. K. (2011). Standards of practice for culturally competent nursing care: 2011 update. *Journal of Transcultural Nursing, 22*(4), 317–333.

Dowsett, S. M., Saul, J. L., Butow, P. N., Dunn, S. M., Boyer, M. J., Findlow, R., & Dunsmore, J. (2000). Communication styles in the cancer consultation: Preferences for a patient-centered approach. *Psychosocial Oncology, 9*(2), 147–156.

Duffield, P. (1998). Advance directives in primary care. *American Journal of Nursing, 98*, 16CCC DDD.

Edmondson, A. C. (1999). Psychological safety and learning behavior in work teams. *Administrative Science Quarterly, 44*, 350–383.

Edmondson, A. C. (2012). *Teaming: How organizations learn, innovate, and compete in the knowledge economy*. A Wiley Imprint.

Eggins S., Geddes F., & Slade D. (Eds.). (2016). *Effective communication in clinical handover – from research to practice (Patient safety, 15)*. De Gruyter Mouton.

Eggins, S., & Slade, D. (2012). Clinical handover as an interactive event: Informational and interactional communication strategies in effective shift-change handovers. *Communication & Medicine, 9*(3), 215.

Eggins, S., & Slade, D. (2015). Communication in clinical handover: Improving the safety and quality of the patient experience. *Journal of Public Health Research, 4*(3), jphr–2015.

Eliott, J., & Olver, I. (2007). Autonomy and the family as (in) appropriate surrogates for DNR decisions: A qualitative analysis of dying cancer patients' talk. *The Journal of Clinical Ethics, 18*(3), 206–218.

Elkılıç, G. (1994). *An analysis of the English language needs of veterinary medicine students at Selçuk* (University Master's thesis, Bilkent University).

Elwyn, G., Edwards, A., Mowle, S., Wensing, M., Wilkinson, C., Kinnersley, P., & Grol, R. (2001). Measuring the involvement of patients in shared decision-making: A systematic review of instruments. *Patient Education and Counseling, 43*(1), 5–22.

Elwyn, G., Laitner, S., Coulter, A., Walker, E., Watson, P., & Thomson, R. (2010). Implementing shared decision making in the NHS. *BMJ, 341*, c5146.

Englar, R. E. (2017). A novel approach to simulation-based education for veterinary medical communication training over eight consecutive pre-clinical quarters. *Journal of Veterinary Medical Education, 44*(3), 502–522.

Englar, R. E. (2019a). Tracking veterinary student progress in clinical communication over eight quarters: A comparison study of the first and final standardized client encounter from the client and student perspective. *Journal of Veterinary Medical Education, 46*(2), 235–257.

Englar, R. E. (2019b). Using a standardized client encounter in the veterinary curriculum to practice veterinarian-employer discussions about animal cruelty reporting. *Journal of Veterinary Medical Education, 45*(4), 464–479.

Englar, R. E. (2019c). Using a standardized client encounter to practice death notification after the unexpected death of a feline patient following routine ovariohysterectomy. *Journal of Veterinary Medical Education, 46*(4), 489–505.

Englar, R. E., Show-Ridgway, A., Noah, D. L., Appelt, E., & Kosinski, R. (2018). Perceptions of the veterinary profession among human health care students before an inter-professional education course at Midwestern University. *Journal of Veterinary Medical Education, 45*(3), 423–436.

Englar, R. E., Williams, M., & Weingand, K. (2016). Applicability of the Calgary–Cambridge guide to dog and cat owners for teaching veterinary clinical communications. *Journal of Veterinary Medical Education, 43*(2), 143–169.

Entwistle, V. A., McCaughan, D., Watt, I. S., Birks, Y., Hall, J., Peat, M., Williams, B., & Wright, J. (2010). Speaking up about safety concerns: Multi-setting qualitative study of patients' views and experiences. *Quality & Safety in Health Care, 19*, e33.

Epner, D. E., & Baile, W. F. (2012). Patient-centered care: The key to cultural competence. *Annals of Oncology: Official Journal of the European Society for Medical Oncology, 23*(Suppl 3), 33–42.

Eppich, W. (2015). "Speaking up" for patient safety in the paediatric emergency department. *Clinical Paediatric Emergency Medicine, 16*(2), 83–89.

Epstein, R. M., Alper, B. S., & Quill, T. E. (2004). Communicating evidence for participatory decision making. *Jama, 291*(19), 2359–2366.

Epstein, R. M., & Street Jr, R. L. (2007). *Patient-centred communication in cancer care: Promoting healing and reducing suffering.* Report, National Cancer Institute.

Erzinger, S. (1991). Communication between Spanish-speaking patients and their doctors in medical encounters. *Culture, Medicine and Psychiatry, 15*(1), 91–110.

Etherington, C., Wu, M., Cheng-Boivin, O., Larrigan, S., & Boet, S. (2019). Interprofessional communication in the operating room: A narrative review to advance research and practice. *Canadian Journal of Anesthesia/Journal Canadien D'anesthésie, 66*(10), 1251–1260.

Evans, D. A., Block, A. R., Steinberg, E. R., & Penrose, A. M. (1986). Frames and heuristics in doctor-patient discourse. *Social Science & Medicine, 22*(10), 1027–1034.

Evans, K. (2015). Emergency departments: Better safe than sorry? *Emergency Nurse, 23*, 20–22.

Evans, S. (2010). Language in transitional Hong Kong: Perspectives from the public and private sectors. *Journal of Multilingual and Multicultural Development, 31*, 347–363.

Evans, W. G., Tulsky, J. A., Back, A. L., & Arnold, R. M. (2006). Communication at times of transitions: How to help patients cope with loss and re-define hope. *The Cancer Journal, 12*(5), 417–424.

Fan, Z., Chen, L., Meng, L, Jiang, H., Zhao, Q., Zhang, L., & Fang, C. (2019). Preference of cancer patients and family members regarding delivery of bad news and differences in clinical practice among medical staff. *Support Care Cancer, 27*(2), 583–589.

Fenton, J. J., Jerant, A. F., Bertakis, K. D., & Franks, P. (2012). The cost of satisfaction: A national study of patient satisfaction, health care utilization, expenditures, and mortality. *Archives of Internal Medicine, 172*(5), 405–411.

Fielding R, Ko L, Wong L, et al (1994). Prevalence and determinants of diagnostic and prognostic disclosure by radiotherapists and surgeons to patients with terminal cancer in Hong Kong. *Journal of the Hong Kong Medical Association*, 46: 220–30.

Fielding, R., & Hung, J. (1996). Preferences for information and involvement in decisions during cancer care among a Hong Kong Chinese population. *Psychooncology, 5*(4), 321–329.

Finnigan, M. A., Marshall, S. D., & Flanagan, B. T. (2010). ISBAR for clear communication: One hospital's experience spreading the message. *Australian Health Review, 34*, 400–404.

Finucane, T. E., & Denman, S. J. (1989). Deciding about resuscitation in a nursing home theory and practice. *Journal of the American Geriatrics Society, 37*, 684–688.

Forde-Johnston, C., Butcher, D., & Aveyard, H. (2023). An integrative review exploring the impact of Electronic Health Records (EHR) on the quality of nurse–patient interactions and communication. *Journal of Advanced Nursing, 79*(1), 48–67.

Frank, R. A. (2000). Medical communication: Non-native English-speaking patients and native English-speaking professionals. *English for Specific Purposes, 19*, 31–62.

Frankel, R. M. (2006). Pets, vets, and frets: What relationship-centered care research has to offer veterinary medicine. *Journal of Veterinary Medicine Education, 33*(1), 20–27.

Frosch, D. L., May, S. G., Rendle, K. A., Tietbohl, C., & Elwyn, G. (2012). Authoritarian physicians and patients' fear of being labeled 'difficult' among key obstacles to shared decision making. *Health Affairs, 31*(5), 1030–1038.

Gaida, S., Härtl, A., Tipold, A., & Dilly, M. (2018). Communication identity in veterinary medicine: A grounded theory approach. *Veterinary Record Open, 5*, 1–11.

García, O. (2009). Education, multilingualism and translanguaging in the 21st century. *Soc Justice Multilingual Education, 143*, 158.

Gelbman, B. D., & Gelbman, J. M. (2008). Deconstructing DNR. *Journal of Medical Ethics, 34*(9), 640–641.

Gillespie, B. M., Gwinner, K., Chaboyer, W., & Fairweather, N. (2013). Team communications in surgery – Creating a culture of safety. *Journal of Interprofessional Care, 27*(5), 387–393.

Glare P. A., & Sinclair, C. T. (2008). Palliative medicine review: Prognostication. *Journal of Palliative Medicine, 11*, 84–103.

Goold, S. D., & Lipkin Jr, M. (1999). The doctor–patient relationship: Challenges, opportunities, and strategies. *Journal of General Internal Medicine, 14*(Suppl 1), S26.

Goto, M., Yokoya, S., Takemura, Y., Gayle, A. A., & Tsuda, T. (2015). Describing the factors that influence the process of making a shared-agenda in Japanese family physician consultations: A qualitative study. *Asia Pacific Family Medicine, 14*(1), 6.

Graffigna, G., Barello, S., Libreri, C., & Bosio, C. A. (2014). How to engage type-2 diabetic patients in their own health management: Implications for clinical practice. *BMC Public Health, 14*, 1–12.

Gramelspacher, G. P., Zhou, X. H., Hanna, M. P., & Tierney, W. M. (1997). Preferences of physicians and their patients for end-of-life care. *Journal of General Internal Medicine, 12*(6), 346–351.

Greenhalgh, T., Robb, N., & Scambler, G. (2006). Communicative and strategic action in interpreted consultations in primary health care: A Habermasian perspective. *Social Science & Medicine, 63*(5), 1170–1187.

Griffiths, S., & Yeoh, E. (2011). *Patient satisfaction survey 2010.*

Gu, Y. G. (1999). A brief introduction to the Chinese health care system. *Health Communication, 11*(3), 203–208.

Gwyn, R., & Elwyn, G. (1999). When is a shared decision not (quite) a shared decision? Negotiating preferences in a general practice encounter. *Social Science & Medicine, 49*(4), 437–447.

Hack, T. F., Degner, L. F., Parker, P. A., & SCRN Communication Team. (2005). The communication goals and needs of cancer patients: A review. *Psychooncology, 14*(10), 831–845.

Haldane, S., Hinchcliff, K., Mansell, P., & Baik, C. (2017). Expectations of graduate communication skills in professional veterinary practice. *Journal of Veterinary Medical Education, 44*, 268–279.

Hamel, M. B., Lynn, J., Teno, J. M., Covinsky, K. E., Wu, A. W., Galanos, A., Desbiens, N. A., & Phillips, R. S. (2000). Age-related differences in care preferences, treatment decisions, and clinical outcomes of seriously ill hospitalized adults: Lessons from SUPPORT. *Journal of the American Geriatrics Society, 48*(S1), S176–S182.

Hamood, W. J., Chur-Hansen, A., & Mcarthur, M. L. (2014). A qualitative study to explore communication skills in veterinary medical education. *International Journal of Medical Science and Education, 5*, 193–198.

Happ, M. B., Garrett, K., Thomas, D. D., Tate, J., George, E., Houze, M., Radtke, J., & Sereika, S. (2011). Nurse-patient communication interactions in the intensive care unit. *American Journal of Critical Care, 20*(2), e28–e40.

Happ, M. B., Tuite, P., Dobbin, K., DiVirgilio-Thomas, D., & Kitutu, J. (2004). Communication ability, method, and content among nonspeaking non-surviving patients treated with mechanical ventilation in the intensive care unit. *American Journal of Critical Care, 13*(3), 210–220.

Härgestam, M., Lindkvist, M., Brulin, C., Jacobsson, M., & Hutlin, M. (2013). Communication in interdisciplinary teams: Exploring closed-loop communication during in situ trauma team training. *BMJ Open*, *3*, e003525.

Harris, J., Herrel, L., Healy, M., Wancata, L., & Perumalswami, C. (2016). Milestones for the final mile: Interspecialty distinctions in primary palliative care skills training. *Journal of Pain and Symptom Management*, *52*, 345–352. e5.

Healey, A. N., Sevdalis, N., & Vincent, C. A. (2006). Measuring intra-operative interference from distraction and interruption observed in the operating theatre. *Ergonomics*, *49*, 589–604.

Health Canada. (2004). *Interdisciplinary education for collaborative patient-centeredness: Research and findings report*. Health Canada, Montreal.

Hemberg, J. A. V., & Vilander, S. (2017). Cultural and communicative competence in the caring relationship with patients from another culture. *Scandinavian Journal of Caring Sciences*, *31*(4), 822–829.

Henderson, A., & Chien, W. T. (2007). Health beliefs and expectations implicit in decision-making in a Hong Kong Chinese surgical population. *Journal of Clinical Nursing*, *16*(3), 603–609.

Henderson, S., Horne, M., Hills, R., & Kendall, E. (2018). Cultural competence in healthcare in the community: A concept analysis. *Health & Social Care in the Community*, *26*(4), 590–603.

Heritage, J., & Maynard, D. W. (Eds.). (2006). *Communication in medical care: Interaction between primary care physicians and patients* (Vol. 20). Cambridge University Press.

Hickmann, E., Richter, P., & Schlieter, H. (2022). All together now–patient engagement, patient empowerment, and associated terms in personal healthcare. *BMC Health Services Research*, *22*(1), 1116.

Ho, E. Y., & Koenig, C. J. (2014). Provider-patient communication about complementary and alternative medicine. In H. E. Hamilton & W. Y. S. Chou (Eds.), *The Routledge handbook of language and health communication* (pp. 506–519). Routledge.

Ho, J. C. Y., Chai, H. H., Lo, E. C. M., Huang, M. Z., & Chu, C. H. (2024). Strategies for effective dentist-patient communication: A literature review. *Patient Preference and Adherence*, 18, 1385–1394.

Holcomb, J., Ferguson, G. M., Thornton, L., & Highfield, L. (2022). Development of training curriculum to improve patient communication skills and social support among community health workers. *HLRP: Health Literacy Research and Practice*, *6*(2), e142–e150.

Holloway, R. G., Gramling, R., & Kelly, A. G. (2013). Estimating and communicating prognosis in advanced neurologic disease. *Neurology*, *80*(8), 764–772.

Hong Kong Hospital Authority. (2013). *Vision, missions & values*.

Hong Kong Hospital Authority. (2014). *Annual report on sentinel and serious untoward events*.

Hong Kong Society of Critical Care Medicine. (2010). *Hong Kong society of critical care medicine's ICU communication board in traditional Chinese.*

Hsiao, F. H., Klimidis, S., Minas, H., & Tan, E. S. (2006). Cultural attribution of mental health suffering in Chinese societies: The views of Chinese patients with mental illness and their caregivers. *Journal of Clinical Nursing, 15*(8), 998–1006.

Hsieh, E., Pitaloka, D., & Johnson, A. J. (2013). Bilingual health communication: Distinctive needs of providers from five specialties. *Health Communication, 28*(6), 557–567.

Hsu, C., O'Connor, M., & Lee, S. (2009). Understandings of death and dying for people of Chinese origin. *Death Studies, 33*(2), 153–174.

Hu, Y. Y., Arriaga, A. F., Peyre, S. E., et al. (2012). Deconstructing intraoperative communication failures. *The Journal of Surgical Research, 177*, 37–42.

Huang, S. C. C., Morgan, A., Peck, V., & Khoury, L. (2021). Improving communications with patients and families in geriatric care. The how, when, and what. *Journal of Patient Experience, 8*, 23743735211034047.

Hudelson, P. (2005). Improving patient–provider communication: Insights from interpreters. *Family Practice, 22*(3), 311–316.

Hudelson, P., & Vilpert, S. (2009). Overcoming language barriers with foreign-language speaking patients: A survey to investigate intra-hospital variation in attitudes and practices. *BioMed Central Health Services Research, 9*, 187.

Hunink, M. M., Weinstein, M. C., Wittenberg, E., Drummond, M. F., Pliskin, J. S., Wong, J. B., & Glasziou, P. P. (2014). *Decision making in health and medicine: Integrating evidence and values*. Cambridge University Press.

Hymes, D. (1964). Introduction: Toward ethnographies of communication 1. *American Anthropologist, 66*(6_PART2), 1–34.

Im, J., Mak, S., Upshur, R., et al. (2019). "Whatever happens, happens" challenges of end-of-life communication from the perspective of older adults and family caregivers: A Qualitative study. *BMC Palliative Care, 18*, 113.

Inman L. (2002). Advance directives: Why community-based older adults do not discuss their wishes. *Journal of Gerontological Nursing, 28*, 40–46.

Institute of Medicine Committee on Quality of Health Care in America. (Eds.). (2001). *Crossing the quality chasm: A new health system for the 21st century.* National Academies Press.

Irvine, F. E., Roberts, G. W., Jones, P., Spencer, L. H., Baker, C. R., & Williams, C. (2006). Communicative sensitivity in the bilingual healthcare setting: A qualitative study of language awareness. *Journal of Advanced Nursing, 53*, 422–434.

Ishikawa, H., & Yamazaki, Y. (2005). How applicable are western models of patient-physician relationship in Asia? Changing patient-physician relationship in contemporary Japan. *International Journal of Japanese Sociology, 14*(1), 84–93.

Iversen, E. D., Wolderslund, M. O., Kofoed, P. E., Gulbrandsen, P., Poulsen, H., Cold, S., & Ammentorp, J. (2020). Codebook for rating clinical communication skills based on the Calgary-Cambridge Guide. *BMC Medical Education, 20*, 1–9.

Jagosh, J., Boudreau, J. D., Steinert, Y., MacDonald, M. E., & Ingram, L. (2011). The importance of physician listening from the patients' perspective: Enhancing diagnosis, healing, and the doctor–patient relationship. *Patient Education and Counseling, 85*(3), 369–374.

Jiang, L. L., Ruan, H., Xiang, X. J., & Jia, Q. (2015). Investigation and analysis of the caring attitude and behaviour of nurses in Shanghai, China. *International Journal of Nursing Practice, 21*(4), 426–432.

Jin, X. W., Slomka, J., & Blixen, C. E. (2002). Cultural and clinical issues in the care of Asian patients. *Cleveland Clinic Journal of Medicine, 69*(1), 50–58.

Jin, Y. (2018). Small talk in medical conversations: Data from China. *Journal of Pragmatics, 134*, 31–44.

Jin, Y. (2022). *Doctor–patient communication in Chinese and western medicine*. Routledge.

Jin, Y., & Tay, D. (2017). Comparing doctor-elderly patient communication between traditional Chinese medicine and Western medicine encounters: Data from China. *Communications Medicine, 14*(2), 121–134.

Joint Commission on Accreditation of Healthcare Organizations. (1998). *Sentinel events: Evaluating cause and planning improvement*. Oakbrook Terrace.

Kaba, R., & Sooriakumaran, P. (2007). The evolution of the doctor-patient relationship. *International Journal of Surgery, 5*(1), 57–65.

Kachalia, A., Gandhi, T. K., Puopolo, A. L., Yoon, C., Thomas, E. J., Griffey, R., Brennan, T. A., & Studdert, D. M. (2007). Missed and delayed diagnoses in the emergency department: A study of closed malpractice claims from 4 liability insurers. *Annals of Emergency Medicine, 49*, 196–205.

Kanaan, R., Armstrong D., & Wessely, S. (2009). Limits to truth-telling: Neurologists' communication in conversion disorder. *Patient Education and Counseling, 77*, 296–301.

Kastbom, L., Karlsson, M., Falk, M., et al. (2020). Elephant in the room-family members' perspectives on advance care planning. *Scandinavian Journal of Primary Health Care, 38*, 421–429.

Katz, M. G., Jacobson, T. A., Veledar, E., & Kripalani, S. (2007). Patient literacy and question-asking behavior during the medical encounter: A mixed-methods analysis. *Journal of General Internal Medicine, 22*, 782–786.

Kee, J. W., Khoo, H. S., Lim, I., & Koh, M. Y. (2018). Communication skills in patient-doctor interactions: Learning from patient complaints. *Health Professions Education, 4*(2), 97–106.

Keeley, M. P. (2016). Family communication at the end of life. *Journal of Family Communication, 16*, 189–197.

Kemp, R., David, A., & Hayward, P. (1996). Compliance therapy: An intervention targeting insight and treatment adherence in psychotic patients. *Behavioural and Cognitive Psychotherapy, 24*(4), 331–350.

Kernick, L. A., Hogg, K. J., Millerick, Y., Murtagh, F. E., Djahit, A., & Johnson, M. (2018). Does advance care planning in addition to usual care reduce hospitalisation for patients with advanced heart failure: A systematic review and narrative synthesis. *Palliative Medicine, 32*(10), 1539–1551.

Kessels, R. P. (2003). Patients' memory for medical information. *Journal of the Royal Society of Medicine, 96*(5), 219–222.

Khalaila, R., Zbidat, W., Anwar, K., Bayya, A., Linton, D. M., & Sviri, S. (2011). Communication difficulties and psychoemotional distress in patients receiving mechanical ventilation. *American Journal of Critical Care, 20*(6), 470–479.

Kim, M., & Oh, S. (2016). Assimilating to hierarchical culture: A grounded theory study on communication among clinical nurses. *PLoS ONE, 11*(6), e0156305.

Kim, S. H., Lee, Y. M., & Park, J. T. (2008). Patients' perspectives on sexual history taking in Korea. *Patient Education and Counseling, 70*(3), 370–375.

Kinnison, T., Guile, D., & May, S. A. (2015). Errors in veterinary practice: Preliminary lessons for building better veterinary teams. *Veterinary Record, 177*(19), 492.

Kitney, P., Tam, R., Bennett, P., et al. (2016). Handover between anaesthetists and post-anaesthetic care unit nursing staff using ISBAR principles: A quality improvement study. *ACORN: The Journal of Perioperative Nursing in Australia, 29,* 30–35.

Klein, B. C., & Busis, N. A. (2020). COVID-19 is catalyzing the adoption of teleneurology. *American Academy of Neurology, 94*(21), 903–904.

Ko, E., & Lee, J. (2009). End-of-life communication: Ethnic differences between Korean American and non-Hispanic white older adults. *Journal of Aging & Health, 21*(7), 967–984.

Ko, E., Roh, S., & Higgins, D. (2003). Do older Korean immigrants engage in end-of-life communication? *Educational Gerontology, 39,* 613–622.

Koehn, P. H., & Swick, H. M. (2006). Medical education for a changing world: Moving beyond cultural competence into transnational competence. *Academic Medicine, 81*(6), 548–556.

Koenig, C. J., Ho, E. Y., Yadegar, V., & Tarn, D. M. (2012). Negotiating complementary and alternative medicine use in primary care visits with older patients.*Patient Education and Counseling, 89*(3), 368–373.

Kogan, L. R., Butler, C. L., Lagoni, L. K., Brannan, J. K., Mcconnell, S. M., & Harvey, A. M. (2004). Training in client relations and communication skills in veterinary medical curricula and usage after graduation. *Journal of the American Veterinary Medical Association, 224,* 504–507.

Konishi, E., & Davis, A. J. (1999). Japanese nurses' perceptions about disclosure of information at the patients' end of life. *Nursing & Health Sciences, 1*(3), 179–187.

Konishi, E., Yahiro, M., Nakajima, N., & Ono, M. (2009). The Japanese value of harmony and nursing ethics. *Nursing Ethics, 16*(5), 625–636.

Kourkouta, L., & Papathanasiou, I. V. (2014). Communication in nursing practice. *Materia Socio-Medica, 26*(1), 65–67.

Kress, H. G., Aldington, D., Alon, E., Coaccioli, S., Collett, B., Coluzzi, F., ... & Sichère, P. (2015). A holistic approach to chronic pain management that involves all stakeholders: Change is needed. *Current Medical Research and Opinion, 31*(9), 1743–1754.

Kress, J. P., Pohlman, A. S., O'Connor, M. F., & Hall, J. B. (2000). Daily interruption of sedative infusions in critically ill patients undergoing mechanical ventilation. *New England Journal of Medicine, 342*(20), 1471–1477.

Kripalani, S., LeFevre, F., Phillips, C. O., William, M. V., Basaviah, P., & Baker D. W. (2007). Deficits in communication and information transfer between hospital-based and primary care physicians: Implications for patient safety and continuity of care. *Jama, 297*, 831–841.

Kurtz, S. (2006). Teaching and learning communication in veterinary medicine. *Journal of Veterinary Medical Education, 33*(1), 11–19.

Kurtz, S. M., & Silverman, J. D. (1996). The Calgary-Cambridge referenced observation guides: An aid to defining the curriculum and organizing the teaching in communication training programmes. *Medical Education, 30*(2), 83–89.

Kurtz, S., Draper, J., & Silverman, J. (2017). *Teaching and learning communication skills in medicine*. CRC Press.

Kvedar, J., Coye, M. J., & Everett, W. (2014). Connected health: A review of technologies and strategies to improve patient care with telemedicine and telehealth. *Health Affairs, 33*(2), 194–199.

Kwak, J., & Haley, W. E. (2005). Current research findings on end-of-life decision making among racially or ethnically diverse groups. *Gerontologist, 45*, 634–641.

Kwak, J., & Salmon, J. R. (2007). Attitudes and preferences of Korean-American older adults and caregivers on end-of-life care. *Journal of the American Geriatrics Society, 55*, 1867–1872.

Lalonde, C., & Adler, C. (2015). Information asymmetry in process consultation: An empirical research on leader-client/consultant relationship in healthcare organizations. *Leadership & Organization Development Journal, 36*(2), 177–211.

Lam, W., Wong, F. Y., & Chan, A. E. (2020). Factors affecting the levels of satisfaction with nurse-patient communication among oncology patients. *Cancer Nursing, 43*(4), E186–E196.

Lamont, E. B., & Christakis, N. A. (2001). Prognostic disclosure to patients with cancer near the end of life. *Annals of Internal Medicine, 134*, 1096–1105.

Landau, R. E., Beck, A., Glickman, L. T., Litster, A., Widmar, N. J. O., & Moore, G. E. (2015). Survey of US veterinary students on communicating with limited English proficient Spanish-speaking pet owners. *Journal of Veterinary Medical Education, 42*, 324–331.

Larson, E. B., & Yao, X. (2005). Clinical empathy as emotional labor in the patient-physician relationship. *Jama, 293*(9), 1100–1106.

Law, B. Y., & Chan, E. A. (2015). The experience of learning to speak up: A narrative inquiry on newly graduated registered nurses. *Journal of Clinical Nursing, 24*, 1837–1848.

Leathart, A. J. (1994). Communication and socialization (1): An exploratory study and explanation for nurse-patient communication in an ITU. *Intensive and Critical Care Nursing, 10*, 93–104.

Lee, J. H., Choi, Y. J., Lee, S. H., Sung, N. J., Kim, S. Y., & Hong, J. Y. (2013). Association of the length of doctor-patient relationship with primary care quality in seven family practices in Korea.*Journal of Korean Medical Science, 28*(4), 508–515.

Lee, S. J., Back, A. L., Block, S. D., & Stewart, S. K. (2002). Enhancing physician-patient communication. *ASH Education Program Book, 2002*(1), 464–483.

Leonard, M., Graham, S., & Bonacum, D. (2004). The human factor: The critical importance of effective teamwork and communication in providing safe care. *Quality & Safety in Health Care, 13*(1), i85–i90.

Leung, C. C. H., Pun, J., Lock, G., Slade, D., Gomersall, C. D., Wong, W. T., & Joynt, G. M. (2018). Exploring the scope of communication content of mechanically ventilated patients. *Journal of Critical Care, 44*, 136–141.

Levinson, W., Lesser, C. S., & Epstein, R. M. (2010). Developing physician communication skills for patient-centered care. *Health Affairs, 29*(7), 1310–1318.

Levinson, W., & Roter, D. (1993). The effects of two continuing medical education programs on communication skills of practicing primary care physicians. *Journal of General Internal Medicine, 8*(6), 318–324.

Li, C., Son, N., Abdulkerim, B. A., Jordan, C. A., & Son, C. G. E. (2017). Overcoming communication barriers to healthcare for culturally and linguistically diverse patients. *North American Journal of Medicine and Science, 10*(3), 1967–1977..

Li, E. S. (2015). *Language, society and culture in Hong Kong*. Open University of Hong Kong Press.

Liddle, P. F., Barnes, T. R. E., Curson, D. A., and Patel, M. (1993). Depression and the experience of psychological deficits in schizophrenia. *Acta Psychiatrica Scandinavica, 88*, 243–247.

Lin, M. L., Huang, C. T., & Chen, C. H. (2016). Reasons for family involvement in elective surgical decision-making in Taiwan: A qualitative study. *Journal of Clinical Nursing, 26*(13–14), 1967–1977.

Lingard L, Espin, S., Whyte, S., et al. (2004). Communication failures in the operating room: An observational classification of recurrent types and effects. *Quality & Safety in Health Care, 13*, 330–334.

Liu, C. H., Tang, W. R., Wang, H. M., & Lee, K. C. (2013). How cancer patients build trust in traditional Chinese medicine. *European Journal of Integrative Medicine, 5*(6), 495–500.

Liu, J. E., Mok, E., & Wong, T. (2005). Caring in nursing: Investigating the meaning of caring from the perspective of cancer patients in Beijing, China. *Journal of Clinical Nursing, 15*, 188–196.

Lo, R. S., Woo, J., Zhoc, K. C., et al. (2001). Cross-Cultural validation of the McGill quality of life questionnaire in Hong Kong Chinese. *Palliative Medicine, 15*, 387–397.

LoPresti, M. A., Dement, F., & Gold, H. T. (2016). End-of-life care for people with cancer from ethnic minority groups: A systematic review. *American Journal of Hospice and Palliative Medicine, 33*(3), 291–305.

Lorié, Á., Reinero, D. A., Phillips, M., Zhang, L., & Riess, H. (2017). Culture and nonverbal expressions of empathy in clinical settings: A systematic review. *Patient Education and Counseling, 100*(3), 411–424.

Lornark, T., & Muangsamai, P. (2010). Needs for and problems about academic English reading of veterinary undergraduate students at Kasetsart university. *Manutsayasat Wichakan, 17*, 165–178.

Low, J. A., Kiow, S. L., Main, N., et al. (2009). Reducing collusion between family members and clinicians of patients referred to the palliative care team. The *Permanente Journal, 13*, 11–15.

Lu, A. P., Jia, H. W., Xiao, C., & Lu, Q. P. (2004). Theory of traditional Chinese medicine and therapeutic method of diseases. *World Journal of Gastroenterology, 10*(13), 1854.

Lum, H. D., Sudore, R. L., & Bekelman, D. B. (2015). Advance care planning in the elderly. *Medical Clinics, 99*(2), 391–403.

Luong, J., Yoder, M. K., & Canham, D. (2009). Southeast Asian parents raising a child with autism: A qualitative investigation of coping styles. *The Journal of School Nursing, 25*, 222–229.

Lyndon, A., Sexton, J. B., Simpson, K. R., Rosenstein, A., Lee, K. A., & Wachter, R. M. (2012). Predictors of likelihood of speaking up about safety concerns in labour and delivery. *BMJ Quality & Safety, 21*(9), 791–709.

Maguire, P. (1990). Can communication skills be taught? *British Journal of Hospital Medicine, 43*(3), 215–216.

Mak, M. H. J. (2001). Awareness of dying: An experience of Chinese patients with terminal cancer. *Omega, 43*(3), 259–279.

Mak, W. W., Cheung, F. M., Wong, S. Y., Tang, W. K., Lau, J. T., Woo, J., & Lee, D. T. (2015). Stigma towards people with psychiatric disorders. *Hong Kong Medical Journal, 21*(Suppl 2), 9–12.

Makary, M. A., Sexton, J. B., Freischlag, J. A., Millman, E. A., Pryor, D., Holzmueller, C., & Pronovost, P. J. (2006). Patient safety in surgery. *Annals of Surgery, 243*(5), 628–635.

Makoul, G. (2001). Essential elements of communication in medical encounters: The Kalamazoo consensus statement. *Academic Medicine, 76*(4), 390–393.

Martini, J. (2018). Patient-provider communication and interactions. In T. P. Daaleman & M. R. Helton (Eds.), *Chronic illness care: Principles and practice* (pp. 187–197). Springer.

Maschler, Y. (1998). On the transition from code-switching to a mixed code. In P. Auer (Eds.), *Code-switching in conversation: language, interaction and identity* (pp. 125–149). Routledge.

Matthiessen, C. M. I. M. (2013). Applying systemic functional linguistics in healthcare contexts. *Text and Talk, 33*, 437–466.

Mauranen, A. (2006). Signaling and preventing misunderstanding in English as lingua franca communication. *International Journal of the Sociology of Language, 2006*(177), 123–150.

Maxwell, H. M. (2018). *The impact of misdiagnosis on psychological well-being: Lessons from Celiac disease.* John F. Kennedy University.

Maynard, D. W., & Heritage, J. (2005). Conversation analysis, doctor-patient interaction and medical communication. *Medical Education, 39*(4), 428–435.

McDarby, M., Picchiello, M., & Kozlov, E. K. (2019). Adult children's understanding of parents' care and living preferences at end of life. *Innovation in Aging, 3*(Suppl 1), S668–9.

Mcdermott, M. P., Tischler, V. A., Cobb, M. A., Robbé, I. J., & Dean, R. S. (2015). Veterinarian-client communication skills: Current state, relevance, and opportunities for improvement. *Journal of Veterinary Medical Education, 42*, 305–314.

McGrath, P., Vun, M., & McLeod, L. (2001). Needs and experiences of non-English-speaking hospice patients and families in an English-speaking country. *The American Journal of Hospice & Palliative Car, 18*(5), 305–312.

Mclaughlin, S., Fitch, M. T., Goyal, D. G., Hayden, E., Kauh, C. Y., Laack, T. A., et al. (2008). Simulation in graduate medical education 2008: A review for emergency medicine. *Academic Emergency Medicine, 15*(11), 1117–1129.

Mechanic, D., & Meyer, S. (2000). Concepts of trust among patients with serious illness. *Social Science & Medicine, 51*(5), 657–668.

Mechanic, D., & Schlesinger, M. (1996). The impact of managed care on patients' trust in medical care and their physicians. *Jama, 275*(21), 1693–1697.

Mehta, A., Najjar, S., May, N., Shah, B., & Blackhall, L. (2018). A needs assessments of palliative care education among the United States adult neurology resident programs.*Journal of Palliative Medicine, 21*, 1448–1457.

Menzel, L. (1998). Factors related to the emotional responses of intubated patients to being unable to speak. *Heart & Lung, 27*, 245–252.

Mesmer-Magnus, J. R., & DeChurch, L. A. (2009). Information sharing and team performance: A meta-analysis. *Journal of Applied Psychology, 94*, 535–546.

Miljeteig, I., Johansson, K. A., Sayeed, S. A., et al. (2010). End-Of-Life decisions as bedside rationing. An ethical analysis of life support restrictions in an Indian neonatal unit.*Journal of Medical Ethics, 36*, 473–478.

Mills, P., Neily, J., & Dunn, E. (2008). Teamwork and communication in surgical teams: Implications for patient safety. *Journal of the American College of Surgeons, 206*(1), 107–112.

Morgan, H. M., Entwistle, V. A., Cribb, A., Christmas, S., Owens, J., Skea, Z. C., & Watt, I. S. (2017). We need to talk about purpose: A critical interpretive synthesis of health and social care professionals' approaches to self-management support for people with long-term conditions. *Health Expectations, 20*(2), 243–259.

Morrison, E. W., & Milliken, F. J. (2003). Speaking up, remaining silent: The dynamics of voice and silence in organizations. *Journal of Management Studies, 40*, 1353–1358.

Mudiyanse, R. M. (2016). Empathy for patient centeredness and patient empowerment. *Journal of General Practice*, *4*(1), 224.

Mullick, A., Martin, J., & Sallnow, L. (2013). An introduction to advance care planning in practice. *BMJ (Clinical research ed.)*, *347*, f6064.

Myhren, H., Toien, K., Ekeberg, O., Karlsson, S., Sandvik, L., & Stokland, O. (2009). Patients' memory and psychological distress after ICU stay compared with expectations of the relatives. *Intensive and Critical Care Nursing*, *35*(12), 2078–2086.

Nápoles-Springer, A. M., Santoyo, J., Houston, K., Pérez-Stable, E. J., & Stewart, A. L. (2005). Patients' perceptions of cultural factors affecting the quality of their medical encounters. *Health Expectations: An International Journal of Public Participation in Health Care and Health Policy*, *8*(1), 4–17.

National Consortium of Telehealth Resource Centers. (2019). *NCTRC webinar–telemedicine: How to do it right*!

Nedjat-Haiem, F. R., Carrion, I. V., Lorenz, K. A., Ell, K., & Palinkas, L. (2013). Psychosocial concerns among Latinas with life-limiting advanced cancers. *Omega*, *67*(1–2), 167–174.

Newham, G. M., Burns, W. I., Snyder, R. D., et al. (2006). Information from the internet: Attitudes of Australian oncology patients. *Internal Medicine Journal*, *36*, 718–723.

Ng, G. W. Y., Pun, J. K. H., So, E. H. K., et al. (2017a). Speak-up culture in an intensive care unit in Hong Kong: A cross-sectional survey exploring the communication openness perceptions of Chinese doctors and nurses, *BMJ Open*, *7*, e015721.

Ng, G. W. Y., Pun, J, So, E. H. K., Chiu, W. W. H., Leung, A. S. H., Stone, Y. H., Lam, C. L., Lai, S. P. W., Leung, R. P. W., Luk, H. W., Leung, A. K. H., Au-Yeung, K. W., Lai, K. Y., Slade, D., & Chan, E. A. (2017b). Exploring speaking-up culture in an intensive care unit (ICU): Chinese doctors' and nurses' perceptions of the openness of communication. *BMJ Open*, *7*(8), 420–430.

Nogueira, B. L. J., Adams, C. L., & Ladner, L. D. (2008). The use of standardized clients in research in the veterinary clinical setting. *Journal of Veterinary Medical Education*, *35*(3), 420–430.

Noh, H. I., Lee, J. M., Yun, Y. H., Park, S. Y., Bae, D. S., Nam, N. J., et al. (2009). Cervical cancer patient information-seeking behaviours, information needs, and information sources in South Korea. *Support. Care Cancer*, *17*(10), 1277–1283.

Nolan, T. W. (2000). System changes to improve patient safety. *BMJ*, *320*, 771–773.

Norals, T. E., & Smith, T. J. (2015). Advance care planning discussions: Why they should happen, why they don't, and how we can facilitate the process. *Oncology*, *29*(8), 567.

Nouri, S. S., Barnes, D. E., Volow, A. M., McMahan, R. D., Kushel, M., Jin, C., et al. (2019). Health literacy matters more than experience for advance care planning knowledge among older adults. *Journal of the American Geriatrics Society*, *67*, 2151–2156.

Nutbeam, D. (2000). Health literacy as a public health goal: A challenge for contemporary health education and communication strategies into the 21st century. *Health Promotion International*, *15*, 259–267.

O'Daniel, M., & Rosenstein, A. H. (2008). Professional communication and team collaboration. In R. G. Hughes (Ed.), *Patient safety and quality: An evidence-based handbook for nurses* (Chapter 33). Agency for Healthcare Research and Quality.

Odgers, J., Fitzpatrick, D., & Penney, W. (2018). No one said he was dying: Families' experiences of end-of-life care in an acute setting. *Australian Journal of Advanced Nursing, 35*, 21.

Ohtaki, S., Ohtaki, T., & Fetters, M. D. (2003). Doctor–patient communication: A comparison of the USA and Japan. *Family Practice, 20*(3), 276–282.

Ong, L. M., Visser, M. R., Lammes, F. B., & De Haes, J. C. (2000). Doctor-patient communication and cancer patients' quality of life and satisfaction. *Patient Education and Counseling, 41*(2), 145–156.

Ong, R. (2023). Factors affecting patient and public perceptions of the adoption of electronic health record sharing: A Hong Kong study. *International Journal of Medical Informatics, 178*, 105193.

Osborne-Smith, L., & Hodgen, R. K. (2017). Communication in the operating room setting. *Annual Review of Nursing Research, 35*, 55–69.

Østbye, T., Yarnall, K. S., Krause, K. M., Pollak, K. I., Gradison, M., & Michener, J. L. (2005). Is there time for management of patients with chronic diseases in primary care? *The Annals of Family Medicine, 3*(3), 209–214.

Park, S. Y., Phua, J., Nishimura, M., Deng, Y., Kang, Y., Tada, K., & Koh, Y. (2018). End-of-life care in ICUs in East Asia: A comparison among China, Korea, and Japan. *Critical Care Medicine, 46*(7), 1114–1124.

Parkinson's Community Help. (2022). 'Managing your healthcare: Communication between the primary care doctor and neurologist' – Webinar notes. *Stanford PD Community Blog.*

Patak, L., Gawlinski, A., Fung, N. I., Doering, L., & Berg, J. (2004). Patients' reports of health care practitioner interventions that are related to communication during mechanical ventilation. *Heart & Lung, 33*(5), 308–320.

Patak, L., Gawlinski, A., Fung, N. I., Doering, L., Berg, J., & Henneman, E. A. (2006). Communication boards in critical care: Patients' views. *Applied Nursing Research, 19*(4), 182–190.

Paternotte, E., van Dulmen, S., van der Lee, N., Scherpbier, A. J., & Scheele, F. (2015). Factors influencing intercultural doctor–patient communication: A realist review. *Patient Education and Counseling, 98*(4), 420–445.

Pawelek, J., Baca-Motes, K., Pandit, J. A., Berk, B. B., & Ramos, E. (2022). The power of patient engagement with electronic health records as research participants. *JMIR Medical Informatics, 10*(7), e39145.

Pearse, W., Saxon, R., Plowman, G., Hyde, M., & Oprescu, F. (2021). Continuing education outcomes for advance care planning: A systematic review of the literature. *Journal of Continuing Education in the Health Professions, 41*(1), 39–58.

Pendleton, D., Schofield, T., Tate, P., & Havelock, P. (2003). *The new consultation: Developing doctor-patient communication*. Oxford University Press.

Peng, N. H., Liu, H. L., Chen, C. H., et al. (2012). Cultural practices and end-of-life decision making in the neonatal intensive care unit in Taiwan. *Journal of Transcultural Nursing, 23*, 320–326.

Pepper, E., Mohan, A., Butcher, K., Parsons, M., & Curtis, J. (2022). Functional neurological disorders: An Australian interdisciplinary perspective. *The Medical Journey of Australis, 216*(10), 501–503.

Periyakoil, V. S., Neri, E., & Kraemer, H. C. (2015). No easy talk: A mixed methods study of doctor reported barriers to conducting effective end-of-life conversations with diverse patients. *PLoS One, 10*, e0122321.

Pezzolesi, C., Schifano, F., Pickles, J., Randell, W., Hussain, Z., Muir, H., & Dhillon, S. (2010). Clinical handover incident reporting in one UK general hospital. *International Journal for Quality in Health Care, 22*(5), 396–401.

Piers, R., Albers, G., Gilissen, J., De Lepeleire, J., Steyaert, J., Van Mechelen, W., ... & Van den Block, L. (2018). Advance care planning in dementia: Recommendations for healthcare professionals. *BMC Palliative Care, 17*, 1–17.

Pinelli, V., Stuckey, H. L., & Gonzalo, J. D. (2017). Exploring challenges in the patient's discharge process from the internal medicine service: A qualitative study of patients' and providers' perceptions. *Journal of Interprofessional Care, 31*(5), 566–574.

Ptacek, J. T., Fries, E. A., Eberhardt, T. L., & Ptacek, J. J. (1999). Breaking bad news to patients: Physicians' perceptions of the process. *Support Care Cancer, 7*(3), 113–120.

Pun, J. (2020). Moments of 'touch' as a way for mental support in Traditional Chinese Medicine consultations: Analysis of the interactional process of co-constructing understanding of the patient's body conditions in Hong Kong. *Complementary Therapies in Medicine*, 52 (102516). https://doi.org/10.1016/j.ctim.2020.102516.

Pun, J. (2020a). An ethnographic discourse analysis: Developing a research-informed training program for effective nursing clinical handover communication. In *SAGE Research Methods Cases: Medicine and Health.* SAGE Publications, Ltd.

Pun, J. (2020b). An integrated review of the role of communication in veterinary clinical practice. *BMC Veterinary Research, 16*, 394.

Pun, J. (2020c). Interdisciplinary research. In McKinley, J. & Rose, H. (Eds.), *The Routledge handbook of research methods in applied linguistics* (pp. 108–121). Routledge.

Pun, J. (2020d). Moments of 'touch' as a way for mental support in Traditional Chinese Medicine consultations: Analysis of the interactional process of co-constructing understanding of the patient's body conditions in Hong Kong. *Complementary Therapies in Medicine, 52*, 102516.

Pun, J. (2021). Clinical handover in a bilingual setting: Interpretative phenomenological analysis to exploring translanguaging practices for effective communication among hospital staff. BMJ Open, 11:e046494, 1-9. http://dx.doi.org/10.1136/bmjopen-2020-046494

Pun, J. (2021a). A study of Chinese medical students' communication pattern in delivering bad news: An ethnographic discourse analysis approach. *BMC Medical Education, 21*(286), 1–10.

Pun, J. (2021b). Clinical handover in a bilingual setting: Interpretative phenomenological analysis to exploring translanguaging practices for effective communication among hospital staff. *BMJ Open, 11*, e046494.

Pun, J. (2021c). Comparing veterinary students' and practitioners' perceptions of communication in a bilingual context. *Veterinary Record, 189*(12), e587.

Pun, J. (2021d). Factors associated with nurses' perceptions, their communication skills and the quality of clinical handover in the Hong Kong context. *BMC Nursing, 20*(1), 95.

Pun, J. (2022). The priorities, challenges, and scope of clinical communication teaching perceived by clinicians from different disciplines: A Hong Kong case study. *BMC Primary Care, 22*(158), 1–16. https://doi.org/10.1186/s12875-022-01770-3

Pun J. (2023a). Nurses' perceptions of the ISBAR handover protocol and its relationship to the quality of handover: A case study of bilingual nurses. *Frontiers in Psychology, 14*, e1021110.

Pun, J. (2023b). Researching veterinary medicine communication. In J. Pun (Ed.), The role of language in eastern and western health communication (pp. 178–200). Routledge.

Pun, J. (2023c). *The role of language in eastern and western health communication*. Routledge.

Pun, J. (2023d). Developing an ESP workshop to promote handover practices in nursing communication: A case study of nurses in a bilingual hospital in Hong Kong. *English for Specific Purposes, 71*, 123–138.

Pun, J., Chan, E. A., Eggins, S., & Slade, D. (2020a). Training in communication and interaction during shift-to-shift nursing handovers in a bilingual hospital: A case study. *Nurse Education Today, 84*, 104212.

Pun, J., Chan, E. A., Man, M., Eggins, S., & Slade, D. (2019a). Pre-and post evaluations of the effects of the Connect, Ask, Respond and Empathise (CARE) protocol on nursing handover: A case study of a bilingual hospital in Hong Kong. *Journal of Clinical Nursing, 28*(15–16), 3001–3011.

Pun, J., Chan, E. A., Matthiessen C. M. I. M., Slade, D., & Murray, K. (2016a). Clinicians' perceptions of communication challenges in a trilingual emergency department in Hong Kong. *Journal of Clinical Nursing, 26*(21–22), 3396–3407.

Pun, J., Chan, E. A., Matthiessen, C. M. I. M., Willian, G., Espindola, E., Veloso, F., Tsui, K. L., & Tang, K. S. (2015a). Effective healthcare worker-patient communication in Hong Kong accident & emergency department. *Hong Kong Journal Emergency Medicine, 22*(2), 69–83.

Pun, J., Chan, E. A., Wang, S., & Slade, D. (2018). Health professional-patient communication practices in East Asia: An integrative review of an emerging field of research and practice in Hong Kong, South Korea, Japan, Taiwan, and Mainland

China. *Patient Education and Counseling, 101*(7), 1193–1206. https://doi.org/10.1016/j.pec.2018.01.018

Pun, J., Cheung K. M., & Chow, C. H. J. (2021a). A systematic review of teaching end of life communication: The priorities, the challenges and the scope. *BMJ Supportive & Palliative Care, 12*(4), 368–375.

Pun, J., & Chor, W. (2020). Use of questioning between traditional chinese medicine practitioners and patients to realize TCM philosophy: Holism, five elements and yin-yang in the context of doctor–patient communication. *Health Communication, 37*(2), 163–176.

Pun, J., Chor, W., & Zhong, L. (2019). Delivery of patient-centred care in complementary medicine: Insights and evidence from the Chinese medical practitioners and patients in primary care consultations in Hong Kong. *Complementary Therapies in Medicine, 45*, 198–204. https://doi.org/10.1016/j.ctim.2019.06.013.

Pun, J., Chow, J. C. H., Fok, L., & Cheung, K. M. (2023). The role of patients' family members in end-of-life communication: An integrative review. *BMJ Open, 13*(2), e067304.

Pun, J. K. (2020). Moments of 'touch'as a way for mental support in traditional Chinese Medicine consultations: analysis of the interactional process of co-constructing understanding of the patient's body conditions in Hong Kong. *Complementary Therapies in Medicine, 52*, 102516.

Pun, J. K. H., Cheung, K. M., Chow, J. C., & Chan, W. L. (2020). Chinese perspective on end-of-life communication: A systematic review. *BMJ Supportive & Palliative Care,* 48, 55–67. https://doi.org/10.1136/bmjspcare-2019-002166

Pun, J. K. H. (2022). Communication about advance directives and advance care planning in an east asian cultural context: A systematic review. *Oncology Nursing Forum, 49*(1), 55–67.

Pun, J. K. H., Cheung, K. M., & Chow, J. C. H. (2021b). Teaching end-of-life communication: Priorities, challenges, scope—systematic review. *BMJ Supportive & Palliative Care, 12*(4), 368–375.

Pun, J., Matthiessen, C. M. I. M., Slade, D., & Murray, K. (2015). Factors affecting communication in emergency departments: Doctors and nurses' perceptions of communication in a trilingual ED in Hong Kong. *International Journal of Emergency Medicine, 8*, 48. https://doi.org/10.1186/s12245-015-0095-y

Pun, J., Matthiessen, C., Williams, G., & Slade, D. (2017). Using ethnographic discourse analysis to understand doctor-patient interactions in clinical settings. In *SAGE Research Methods Cases*. SAGE Publications, Ltd.

Pun, J., & Wong, W. (2022). Navigating communication between conventional medicine and traditional Chinese medicine: A case study of cancer patients in Hong Kong. *Supportive Care in Cancer, 30*(7), 5729–5735.

Pun, K. H. J., Chan, E. A., Murray, K. A., Slade, D., & Matthiessen, C. M. I. M. (2016b). Complexities of emergency communication: Clinicians' perceptions of communication challenges in a trilingual emergency department. *Journal of Clinical Nursing, 26*(21–22), 3396–3407.

Radford, A. D., Stockley, P., Taylor, I. R., Turner, R., Gaskell, C. J., Kaney, S., et al. (2003). Use of simulated clients in training veterinary undergraduates in communication skills. *Veterinary Record, 152*, 422–427.

Rajkomar, A., Dean, J., & Kohane, I. (2019). Machine learning in medicine. *The New England Journal of Medicine, 380*(14), 1347–1358.

Rattray, N. A., Sico, J. J., Cox, L. M., Russ, A. L., Matthias, M. S., & Frankel, R. M. (2017). Crossing the communication chasm: Challenges and opportunities in transitions of care from the hospital to the primary care clinic. *The Joint Commission Journal on Quality and Patient Safety, 43*(3), 127–137.

Ribeiro B. T., & Hoyle, S. M. (2009). Frame analysis. *Grammar Meaning Pragmatics, 5*, 74.

Rider, E. A., Kurtz, S., Slade, D., Longmaid, E. III. H. E., Ho, M. J., Pun, K. H., Eggins, S. & Branch, W. T. (September 2014) The international charter for human values in healthcare: An interprofessional global collaboration to enhance values and communication in healthcare. *Patient Education and Counseling, 96*(3), 273–280.

Robertson, E. R., Morgan, L., Bird, S., et al. (2014). Interventions employed to improve intrahospital handover: A systematic review. *BMJ Quality & Safety, 23*, 1–8.

Rocque, R., & Leanza, Y. (2015). A systematic review of patients' experiences in communicating with primary care physicians: Intercultural encounters and a balance between vulnerability and integrity. *PloS One, 10*(10), e0139577.

Rogers, P. C., Graham, C. R., & Mayes, C. T. (2007). Cultural competence and instructional design: Exploration research into the delivery of online instruction cross-culturally. *Educational Technology Research and Development, 55*, 197–217.

Rønning, S. B., & Bjørkly, S. (2019). The use of clinical role-play and reflection in learning therapeutic communication skills in mental health education: An integrative review. *Advances in Medical Education and Practice*, 415–425.

Rösch, T., Schaper, E., Tipold, A., Fischer, M. R., Dilly, M., & Ehlers, J. P. (2014). Clinical skills of veterinary students – A cross-sectional study of the self-concept and exposure to skills training in Hannover, Germany. *BMC Veterinary Research, 10*, 969.

Russell, J. (2016). The role of health care provider goals, plans, and physician orders for life sustaining treatment (POLST) in preparing for conversations about end-of-life care. *J HealthCommun, 21*(9), 1023–1030.

Sampson, E. L., Jones, L., Thuné-Boyle, I. C. V., Kukkastenvehmas, R., King, M., Leurent, B., et al. (2011). Palliative assessment and advance care planning in severe dementia: An exploratory randomized controlled trial of a complex intervention.*Palliative Medicine, 25*, 197–209.

Schapira, L. (2006). Delivering bad news to patients and their families. In K. N. Syrigos, C. M. Nutting, & C. Roussos (Eds.), *Tumors of the Chest* (pp. 597–605). Springer.

Schenker, Y., Fernandez, A., Sudore, R, & Schillinger, D. (2011). Interventions to improve patient comprehension in informed consent for medical and surgical procedures: A systematic review. *Medical Decision Making, 31*, 151–173.

Schiff, L., Tsafrir, Z., Aoun, J., Taylor, A., Theoharis, L., & Eisenstein, D. (2016). Quality of communication in robotic surgery and surgical outcomes. *Journal of the Society of Laparoendoscopic Surgeons, 20*(3), e2016.00026.

Schillinger, D., Piette, J., Grumbach, K., Wang, F., Wilson, C., Daher, C., Leong-Grotz, K., Castro, C., & Bindman, A. B. (2003). Closing the loop: Physician communication with diabetic patients who have low health literacy. *Archives of Internal Medicine, 163*(1), 83–90.

Schouten, B. C., & Meeuwesen, L. (2006). Cultural differences in medical communication: A review of the literature. *Patient Education and Counseling, 64*(1–3), 21–34.

Schuenemeyer, J., Hong, Y., Plankey, M., et al. (2017). Foreign body entrapment during thoracic surgery—time for closed loop communication. *European Journal of Cardio-Thoracic Surgery, 51*, 852–855.

Schuh, L. A., Adair, J. C., Drogan, O., Kissela, B. M., Morgenlander, J. C., & Corboy, J. R. (2009). Education research: Neurology residency training in the new millennium. *Neurology, 72*, e15–e20.

Schulz, P. J., & Nakamoto, K. (2013). Health literacy and patient empowerment in health communication: The importance of separating conjoined twins. *Patient Education and Counseling, 90*(1), 4–11.

Schwappach, D. L., & Gehring, K. (2014). Trade-offs between voice and silence: A qualitative exploration of oncology staff's decisions to speak up about safety concerns. *BMC Health Services Research, 14*, 303.

Scott, A. M. (2010). *Family conversations about end-of-life health decisions* (PhD thesis, University of Illinois at Urbana-Champaign).

Scott, A. M., & Caughlin, J. P. (2014). Enacted goal attention in family conversations about end-of-life health decisions. *Communication Monographs, 81*(3), 261–284.

Searight, H. R. (2022). Cross-cultural issues in end-of-life care: A selective overview of recent research and ethical perspectives. *Advances in Sociology Research, 139*.

Seijo, R., Gomez, H., & Freidenberg, J. (1991). Language as a communication barrier in medical care for Hispanic patients. *Hispanic Journal of Behavioral Sciences, 13*(4), 363–376.

Sevdalis, N., Healey, A. N., & Vincent, C. A. (2007). Distracting communications in the operating theatre. *Journal of Evaluation in Clinical Practice, 13*, 390–394.

Shahid, S., & Thomas, S. (2018). Situation, background, assessment, recommendation (SBAR) communication tool for handoff in health care–A narrative review. *Safety in Health, 4*(1), 1–9.

Shaw, J. R., Adams, C. L., & Bonnett, B. N. (2004). What can veterinarians learn from studies of physician-patient communication about veterinarian-client-patient communication? *Journal of the American Veterinary Medical Association, 224*, 676–684.

Shelley, B. M., Sussman, A. L., Williams, R. L., Segal, A. R., & Crabtree, B. F. (2009). 'They don't ask me so I don't tell them': Patient-clinician communication about traditional, complementary, and alternative medicine. *The Annals of Family Medicine*, *7*(2), 139–147.

Shersher, V., Haines, T. P., Sturgiss, L., Weller, C., & Williams, C. (2021). Definitions and use of the teach-back method in healthcare consultations with patients: A systematic review and thematic synthesis. *Patient Education and Counseling*, *104*(1), 118–129.

Shih, T. C., Chang, H. T., Lin, M. H., Chen, C. K., Chen, T. J., & Hwang, S. J. (2017). Trends of do-not-resuscitate orders, hospice care utilization, and late referral to hospice care among cancer decedents in a tertiary hospital in Taiwan between 2008 and 2014: A hospital-based observational study. *Journal of Palliative Medicine*, *20*(8), 838–844.

Show, A., & Englar, R. E. (2018). Evaluating dog-and cat-owner preferences for calgary-cambridge communication skills: Results of a questionnaire. *Journal of Veterinary Medical Education*, *45*(4), 534–543.

Shrank, W. H., Kutner, J. S., Richardson, T., Mularski, R. A., Fischer, S., & Kagawa-Singer, M. (2005). Focus group findings about the influence of culture on communication preferences in end-of-life care. *Journal of General Internal Medicine*, *20*(8), 703–709.

Silva, M. D., Genoff, M., Zaballa, A., et al. (2016). Interpreting at the end of life: A systematic review of the impact of interpreters on the delivery of palliative care services to cancer patients with limited English proficiency. *Journal of Pain & Symptom Management*, *51*(3), 569–580.

Simon, S. R., Evans, J. S., Benjamin, A., Delano, D., & Bates, D. W. (2009). Patients' attitudes toward electronic health information exchange: Qualitative study. *Journal of Medical Internet Research*, *11*(3), e30.

Singh, H., & Dey, A. K. (2021). Listen to my story: Contribution of patients to their healthcare through effective communication with doctors. *Health Services Management Research*, *34*(3), 178–192.

Siu, J. Y. M. (2015). Communicating under medical patriarchy: Gendered doctor-patient communication between female patients with overactive bladder and male urologists in Hong Kong. *BMC Women's Health*, *15*(1), 44.

Slade, D., Manidis, M., McGregor, J., Scheeres, H., Chandler, E., Stein-Parbury, J., ... & Matthiessen, C. M. (2015). *Communicating in hospital emergency departments*. Springer.

Slade, D., Chandler, E., Pun, J., Lam, M., Matthiessen, C. M. I. M., & Williams, G. (2015a). Effective healthcare worker-patient communication in accident and emergency departments. *Hong Kong Journal of Emergency Medicine*, *22*(2), 69–82.

Slade, D., Manidis, M., McGregor, J., Scheeres, H., Chandler, E., Stein-Parbury, J., Dunston, R., Herke, M., & Matthiessen, C. M. I. M. (2015b). *Communicating in hospital emergency departments*. Springer.

Slade, D., Murray, K. A., Pun, J. K., & Eggins, S. (2019). Nurses' perceptions of mandatory bedside clinical handovers: An Australian hospital study. *Journal of Nursing Management, 27*(1), 161171.

Slade, D., Pun, J., Lock, G., & Eggins, S. (2016). Potential risk points in doctor-patient communication: An analysis of Hong Kong emergency department medical consultations. In H. D. S. Joyce (Eds.), *Language at work: Analysing language use in work, education, medical and museum contexts* (pp. 146–165). Cambridge Scholars Publishing.

Slade, D., Pun, J., Murray, K. A., & Eggins, S. (2018). Benefits of health care communication training for nurses conducting bedside handovers: An Australian hospital case study. *The Journal of Continuing Education in Nursing, 49* (7), 329–336.

Smith, R. C., Dorsey, A. M., Lyles, J. S., & Frankel, R. M. (1999). Teaching selfawareness enhances learning about patient-centered interviewing. *Academic Medicine, 74*, 1242–1248.

Smith, S. K., Nutbeam, D., & McCaffery, K. J. (2013). Insights into the concept and measurement of health literacy from a study of shared decision-making in a low literacy population. *Journal of Health & Psychology, 18*, 1011–1122.

Smithers, L. G., Sawyer, A. C., Chittleborough, C. R., Davies, N. M., Davey Smith, G., & Lynch, J. W. (2018). A systematic review and meta-analysis of effects of early life non-cognitive skills on academic, psychosocial, cognitive and health outcomes. *Nature Human Behaviour, 2*, 867–880.

Society of Critical Care Medicine. (2001). *ICU patient communicator app*. http://www.sccm.org/Education-Center/Clinical-Resources/Pages/Patient-and-Family.aspx;

Sørensen, K., Van den Broucke, S., Pelikan, J. M., Fullam, J., Doyle, G., Slonska, Z., et al. (2013). Measuring health literacy in populations: Illuminating the design and development process of the European Health Literacy Survey Questionnaire (HLS-EU-Q). *BMC Public Health, 13*, 1–10.

Sparks, L., Villagran, M. M., Parker-Raley, J., & Cunningham, C. B. (2007). A patient-centered approach to breaking bad news: Communication guidelines for health care providers. *Journal of Applied Communication Research, 35*(2), 177–196.

Squier, R. W. (1990). A model of empathic understanding and adherence to treatment regimens in practitioner-patient relationships. *Social Science & Medicine, 30*(3), 325–339.

Steinhubl, S. R., Muse, E. D., & Topol, E. J. (2015). The emerging field of mobile health. *Science Translational Medicine, 7*(283), 283rv3.

Stern, H. H., Stern, H. H., Tarone, E. E., Stern, H., & Yule, G. (1983). *Fundamental concepts of language teaching: Historical and interdisciplinary perspectives on applied linguistic research*. Oxford University Press.

Stern, J. M., Cendes, F., Gilliam, F., Kwan, P., Ryvlin, P., Sirven, J., Smith, B., Adomas, A., & Walter, L. (2018). Neurologist-patient communication about epilepsy in the United States, Spain, and Germany. *Neurology Clinical Practice, 8*(2), 93–101.

Stewart, A. (1995). Effective physician-patient communication and health outcomes: A review. *CMAJ, 152*(9), 1423.

Stiggelbout, A. M., Van der Weijden, T., De Wit, M. P. T., et al. (2012). Shared decision making: Really putting patients at the centre of healthcare. *BMJ, 344*, e256.

Street Jr, R. L., Makoul, G., Arora, N. K., & Epstein, R. M. (2009). How does communication heal? Pathways linking clinician–patient communication to health outcomes. *Patient Education and Counseling, 74*(3), 295–301.

Stuart, P. (2017). Health literacy: A study of internet-based information on advance directives. *Journal of Nursing Management, 24*, 27.

Sun, Y. Q., Sun, B. F., XM Li, J Zhao, P Zhang. (2011). A qualitative study on the reasons for cancer families choosing whether to inform patient the truth. *The Journal of Medicine and Philosophy, 32* ,77–78.

Sutcliffe, K. M., Lewton, E., & Rosenthal, M. N. (2004). Communication failures: An insidious contributor to medical mishaps. *Academic Medicine, 79*, 186–194.

Takayama, T., Yamazaki, Y., & Katsumata, N. (2001). Relationship between outpatients' perceptions of physicians' communication styles and patients' anxiety levels in a Japanese oncology setting. *Social Science & Medicine, 53*(10), 1335–1350.

Tam, A. Y. B., & Lau, F. (2000). A three-year review of complaints in emergency departments. *Hong Kong Journal of Emergency Medicine, 7*(1), 16–21.

Tang, A. C. Y., Chung, J. W. Y., & Wong, T. K. S. (2012). Validation of a novel traditional Chinese medicine pulse diagnostic model using an artificial neural network. *Evidence-based Complementary and Alternative Medicine, 2012*, 685094.

Tang, S. T., Liu, T., Lai M., Liu, L., Chen, C., & Koong, S. (2006). Congruence of knowledge, experiences, and preferences for disclosure of diagnosis and prognosis between terminally-ill cancer patients and their family caregivers in Taiwan. *Cancer Investigation, 24*(4), 360–366.

Taylor, D. M., Wolfe, R., & Cameron, P. A. (2002). Complaints from emergency department patients largely result from treatment and communication problems. *Emergency Medicine Australas, 14*(1), 43–49.

Tembo, A. C., Higgins, I., & Parker, V. (2015). The experience of communication difficulties in critically ill patients in and beyond intensive care: Findings from a larger phenomenological study. *Intensive and Critical Care Nursing, 31*(3), 171–178.

Ten Hoorn, S., Elbers, P. W., Girbes, A. R., Tuinman, P. R. (2016). Communicating with conscious and mechanically ventilated critically ill patients: A systematic review. *Critical Care, 20*(1), 333.

Thompson, J. E., Collett, L. W., Langbart, M. J., Purcell, N. J., Boyd, S. M., Yurninaga, Y., Ossolinski, G., Susanto, C., & McCornack, A. (2011). Using the ISBAR handover tool in junior medical officer handover: A study in an Australian tertiary hospital. *Postgrad Medical Journal, 87*, 340–344.

Tierney, W. M., Dexter, P. R., Gramelspacher, G. P., et al. (2001). The effect of discussions about advance directives on patients' satisfaction with primary care. *Journal of General Internal Medicine, 16*(1), 32–40.

Tiew L. H., & Creedy D. K. (2010). Integration of spirituality in nursing practice: A literature review. *Singapore Nursing Journal, 37*, 15–22.

Timmins, C. L. (2002). The impact of language barriers on the health care of Latinos in the United States: A review of the literature and guidelines for practice. *Journal of Midwifery & Women's Health, 47*, 80–96.

Toda, Y., Sakamoto, M., Tagaya, A., Takahashi, M., & Davis, A. J. (2015). Patient advocacy: Japanese psychiatric nurses recognizing necessity for intervention. *Nursing Ethics, 22*(7), 765–777.

Tongue, J. R., Epps, H. R., & Forese, L. L. (2005). Communication skills for patient-centered care: Research-based, easily learned techniques for medical interviews that benefit orthopaedic surgeons and their patients. *Journal of Bone and Joint Surgery, 87*(3), 652–658.

Tørring, B., Gittell, J. H., Laursen, M., et al. (2019). Communication and relationship dynamics in surgical teams in the operating room: An ethnographic study. *BMC Health Services Research, 19*, 528.

Troyer, L., & Brady, W. (2020). Barriers to effective EMS to emergency department information transfer at patient handover: A systematic review. *The American Journal of Emergency Medicine, 38*(7), 1494–1503.

Trummer, U. F., Mueller, U. O., Nowak, P., Stidl, T., & Pelikan, J. M. (2006). Does physician–patient communication that aims at empowering patients improve clinical outcome? A case study. *Patient Education and Counseling, 61*(2), 299–306.

Tse, C. Y., Chong, A., & Fok, S. Y. (2003). Breaking bad news: A Chinese perspective. *Palliative Medicine, 17*(4), 339–343.

Tulsky J. A. (2005). Beyond advance directives: Importance of communication skills at the end of life. *Jama, 294*(3), 359–365.

van der Steen, J. T. (2010). Dying with dementia: What we know after more than a decade of research. *Journal of Alzheimer's Disease, 22*, 37–55.

Vasquez, C., & Javier, R. A. (1991). The problem with interpreters: Communicating with Spanish-speaking patients. *Psychiatric Services, 42*, 163–165.

Villagran, M., Goldsmith, J., Wittenberg-Lyles, E., et al. (2010). Creating comfort: A communication-based model for breaking bad news. *Communication Education, 59*, 220–234.

Vincent, C., Young, M., & Phillips, A. (1995). Why do people sue doctors? A study of patients and relatives taking legal action. *Obstetrical & Gynecological Survey, 50*(2), 103–105.

Vincent, C. A., & Coulter, A. (2002). Patient safety: What about the patient? *BMJ Quality & Safety, 11*(1), 76–80.

Vincent, C., Young, M., & Phillips, A. (1995). Why do people sue doctors? A study of patients and relatives taking legal action. *Obstetrical & Gynecological Survey, 50*(2), 103–105.

Vranceanu, A. M., Cooper, C., & Ring, D. (2009). Integrating patient values into evidence-based practice: Effective communication for shared decision-making. *Hand Clinics*, *25*(1), 83–96.

Waitzkin, H. (1984). Doctor-patient communication: Clinical implications of social scientific research. *Jama*, *252*, 2441–2446.

Wang, C. W., & Chan, C. L. (2015). End-of-life care research in Hong Kong: A systematic review of peer-reviewed publications. *Palliative & Supportive Care*, *13*(6), 1711–1720.

Wang, Q. (2010). *Doctor-patient communication and patient satisfaction: A cross-cultural comparative study between China and the US* (Unpublished doctoral dissertation, Purdue University).

Wang, S. Y., Chen, C., Chen, Y., & Huang, H. (2004). The attitude toward truth telling of cancer in Taiwan. *Journal of Psychosomatic Research*, *57*(1), 53–58.

Wang, X., Huang, Y., Radha-Krishna, L., et al. (2016). Role of the nasogastric tube and lingzhi (ganoderma lucidum) in palliative care. *Journal of Pain & Symptom Management*, *51*, 794–799.

Weger Jr, H., Castle Bell, G., Minei, E. M., & Robinson, M. C. (2014). The relative effectiveness of active listening in initial interactions. *International Journal of Listening*, *28*(1), 13–31.

Wenger, N. S., Phillips, R. S., Teno, J. M., Oye, R. K., Dawson, N. V., Liu, H., et al. (2000). Physician understanding of patient resuscitation preferences: Insights and clinical implications. *Journal of the American Geriatrics Society*, *48*(Suppl. 5), S44–S51.

Wessely, S. (1999). "To tell or not to tell": The problem of medically unexplained symptoms. In A. Zeman & L. L. Emanuel (Eds.), *Ethical Dilemmas in Neurology* (pp. 41–53). Saunders.

Westli, H. K., Johnsen, B. H., Eid, J., Rasten, I., & Brattebo ,G. (2010). Teamwork skills, shared mental models, and performance in simulated trauma teams: An independent group design. *Scandinavian Journal of Trauma, Resuscitation and Emergency Medicine*, *18*, 47.

Whelan, G. P., Boulet, J. R., Mckinley, D. W., Norcini, J. J., Van Zanten, M., Hambleton, R. K., et al. (2005). Scoring standardized patient examinations: Lessons learned from the development and administration of the ECFMG clinical skills assessment (CSA®). *Medicine Teachology*, 27(3), 200–206.

Wisnivesky, J. P., Kattan, M., Evans, D., et al. (2009). Assessing the relationship between language proficiency and asthma morbidity among inner-city asthmatics. *Medicine Care*, *47*, 243–249.

Wong-Kim, E., Sun, A., & DeMattos, M. C. (2003) Assessing cancer beliefs in a Chinese immigrant community. *Cancer Control*, *10*, 22–8.

Wong, C. A., Cummings, G. G., & Ducharme, L. (2013). The relationship between nursing leadership and patient outcomes: A systematic review update. *Journal of Nursing Management*, *21*(5), 709–724.

Wong, D. K. K., & Cheung, M. K. (2019). Online health information seeking and eHealth literacy among patients attending a primary care clinic in Hong Kong: A cross-sectional survey. *Journal of Medical Internet Research, 21*(3), e10831.

Wong, S. Y., Lo, S. H., Chan, C. H., Chui, H. S., Sze, W. K., & Tung, Y. (2012). Is it feasible to discuss an advance directive with a Chinese patient with advanced malignancy? A prospective cohort study. *Hong Kong Medical Journal, 18*(3), 178–185.

Wright, A. A., Zhang, B., Ray, A., et al. (2008). Associations between end-of-life discussions, patient mental health, medical care near death, and caregiver bereavement adjustment. *Jama, 300*, 1665–1673.

Wu, A. M., Tang, C. S., & Kwok, T. C. (2002). Death anxiety among Chinese elderly people in Hong Kong. *Journal of Aging and Health, 14*(1), 42–56.

Wu, H. Z., Fang, Z. Q., & Cheng, P. J. (2013). *Fundamentals of traditional Chinese medicine.* World Century Publishing Corporation.

Xiao, S., Wang, L., Edelman, E. J., & Khoshnood, K. (2020). Interpersonal factors contributing to tension in the Chinese doctor–patient–family relationship: A qualitative study in Hunan Province. *BMJ Open, 10*(12), e040743.

Xu, Y., & Davidhizar, R. (2005). Intercultural communication in nursing education: When Asian students and American faculty converge. *The Journal of Nursing Education, 44*(5), 209–215.

Xu, J., & Yang, Y. (2009). Traditional Chinese medicine in the Chinese health care system. *Health policy*, 90(2–3), 133–139.

Yam, B. M., & Rossiter, J. C. (2000). Caring in nursing: perceptions of Hong Kong nurses. Journal of Clinical Nursing (Wiley-Blackwell), 9(2).

Yam, B., Rossiter, J. C., & Cheung, K. (2001). Caring for dying infants: Experiences of neonatal intensive care nurses in Hong Kong. *Journal of Clinical Nursing, 10*(5), 651–659.

Yao, M., Yang, Y., Dong, L., Zhou, L., & Ni, J. (2023). An investigation of the current status of doctor-patient communication skills among neurological residents. *Chinese Journal of Stroke, 18*(8), 966–971.

Ye, K., McD Taylor, D., Knott, J. C., Dent, A., & MacBean, C. E. (2007). Handover in the emergency department: Deficienciesand adverse effects. *Emergency Medicine Australasia, 19*, 433–441.

Yeheskel, A., & Rawal, S. (2019). Exploring the 'patient experience'of individuals with limited English proficiency: A scoping review. *Journal of Immigrant and Minority Health, 21*(4), 853–878.

Yin Choi, M. C., Chu, S. H., Siu, L. L., Tse, A. G., Yuen Wu, J. C., Fung, H., ... & Tong Mok, V. C. (2021). Elderly acceptance of telemedicine use in Hong Kong during and after the COVID-19 pandemic: A cross-sectional cohort survey. *medRxiv*, 29(5), 412–420. https://doi.org/10.1101/2021.07.15.21260346.

Yin, C. P., Hsu, C. W., Kuo, F. Y., & Huang, Y. T. (2012). A study of politeness strategies adopted in pediatric clinics in Taiwan. *Health Communication, 27*(6), 533–545.

Yonashiro-Cho, J., Cote, S., & Enguidanos, S. (2016). Knowledge about and perceptions of advance care planning and communication of Chinese-American older adults. *Journal of the American Geriatrics Society, 64*(9), 1884–1889.

Zager, B. S., & Yancy, M. (2011). A call to improve practice concerning cultural sensitivity in advance directives: A review of the literature. *Worldviews on Evidence-Based Nursing, 8*(4), 202–211.

Zayts, O. A., & Kang, M. A. (2010). Communication in healthcare settings: Interactional perspectives from Asia. *Journal of Asian Pacific Communication, 20*(2), 165–168.

Zayts, O., & Kang, M. A. (2013). Interactional difficulties as a resource for patient participation in prenatal screening consultations in Hong Kong. *Patient Education and Counseling, 92*(1), 38–44.

Zehm, A., Hazeltine, A. M., Greer, J. A., Traeger, L., Nelson-Lowe, M., Brizzi, K., & Jacobsen, J. (2020). Neurology clinicians' views on palliative care communication: "How do you frame this?" *Neurology: Clinical Practice, 10*(5), 1–8.

Zhang, B., Wright, A. A., Huskamp, H. A., Nilsson, M. E., Mciejewski, M. L., Earle, C. C., Block, S. D., Maciejewski, P. K., & Prigerson, H. G. (2009). Health care costs in the last week of life: Associations with end-of-life conversations. *Archives of Internal Medicine, 169*(5), 480–488.

Zhang, Q., & Liu, C. Y. (2010). Status quo of knowing the fact and consent of cancer patients and its strategies. *Chinese Nursing Research, 20*, 471–472.

Zhang, X. Q., & Sleeboom-Faulkner, M. (2011). Tensions between medical professionals and patients in Mainland China. *Cambridge Q Healthc Ethics, 20*(3), 458–465.

Zhang, Y., Su, H., Shang, L., Li, D., Wang, R., Zhang, R., & Xu, Y. (2011). Preferences and perceived involvement in treatment decision making among Chinese patients with chronic hepatitis. *Medicine Decision Making, 31*(2), 245–253.

Zheng, R. S., Guo, Q. H., Dong, F. Q., & Owens, R. G. (2015). Chinese oncology nurses' experience on caring for dying patients who are on their final days: A qualitative study. *International Journal of Nursing Studies, 52*(1), 288–296.

Zhou, L., & Nunes, M. B. (2012). Identifying knowledge sharing barriers in the collaboration of traditional and western medicine professionals in Chinese hospitals: A case study. *Journal of Librarianship & Information Science, 44*(4), 238–248.

Zulman, D. M., Haverfield, M. C., Shaw, J. G., Brown-Johnson, C. G., Schwartz, R., Tierney, A. A., ... & Verghese, A. (2020). Practices to foster physician presence and connection with patients in the clinical encounter. *Jama, 323*(1), 70–81.

Zweibel, N. R., & Cassel, C. K. (1989). Treatment choices at the end of life: A comparison of decisions by older patients and their physician-selected proxies. *The Gerontologist, 29*(5), 615–621.

Index

www.ingramcontent.com/pod-product-compliance
Ingram Content Group UK Ltd.
Pitfield, Milton Keynes, MK11 3LW, UK
UKHW020257051026
15470UKWH00020B/1018

9 781350 298118